SERMs
A Novel Option to Maintain Health in the Postmenopause

Donato Agnusdei
Eli Lilly and Company
Florence
Italy

Juliet Compston
University of Cambridge
School of Clinical Medicine
Addenbrooke's Hospital
Cambridge
UK

MARTIN DUNITZ

First published in the United Kingdom in 2000 by:
Martin Dunitz Ltd
The Livery House
7–9 Pratt Street
London NW1 0AE

Tel: +44 (0)207 482 2202
Fax: +44 (0)207 267 0159
E-mail: info@mdunitz.globalnet.co.uk
Website: http://www.dunitz.co.uk

A CIP record for this book is available from the British Library

ISBN 1-85317-820-9

Distributed in the United States by:
Blackwell Science Inc
Commerce Place, 350 Main Street
Malden MA 02148, USA
Tel: 1 800 215 1000

Distributed in Canada by:
Login Brothers Book Company
324 Salteaux Crescent
Winnipeg, Manitoba R3J 3T2
Canada
Tel: 1 204 224 4068

Distributed in Brazil by:
Ernesto Reichmann Distribuidora de Livros, Ltda
Rua Coronel Marques 335, Tatuape 03440-000
Sao Paulo
Brazil

Composition by Wearset, Boldon, Tyne and Wear
Printed and bound in Italy

Contents

Contributors

Donato Agnusdei
Eli Lilly and Company, Florence, Italy

Olivier A Bruyere
Bone and Cartilage Metabolism Unit
Department of Epidemiology and Public Health
University of Liège, Liège, Belgium

Peter Collins
Department of Cardiology, Royal Brompton Hospital,
London, UK

Juliet Compston
Department of Medicine
University of Cambridge, School of Clinical Medicine,
Addenbrooke's Hospital, Cambridge, UK

Cyrus Cooper
Medical Research Council Environmental Epidemiology Unit
University of Southampton, Southampton General Hospital
Southampton, UK

Rita de Cassia M Dardes
Robert H Lurie Comprehensive Cancer Center, Northwestern University Medical School, Chicago, Illinois, USA

Martina Dören
Department of Family Planing,
King's College Hospital, London, UK

Nicoletta Iori
Eli Lilly Italia, Florence, Italy

V Craig Jordan
Robert H Lurie Comprehensive Cancer Center, Northwestern University Medical School, Chicago, Illinois, USA

Fergus SJ Keating
Rosen Laboratories of the Wynn Institute, Endocrinology and Metabolic Medicine, Imperial College School of Medicine, St Mary's Hospital, London, UK

George GJM Kuiper
Department of Internal Medicine Erasmus University Medical School, Rotterdam, The Netherlands

Nikolay Manassiev
Rosen Laboratories of the Wynn Institute, Endocrinology and Metabolic Medicine, Imperial College School of Medicine, St Mary's Hospital, London, UK

Patrick Neven
Algemene Kliniek St-Jan, Brussels, Belgium

David Purdie
Centre for Metabolic Bone Disease
Hull Royal Infirmary, Hull, UK

Jean-Yves Reginster
Bone and Cartilage Metabolism Unit, Department of Epidemiology and Public Health, University of Liège, Liège, Belgium

John C Stevenson
Rosen Laboratories of the Wynn Institute, Endocrinology and Metabolic Medicine, Imperial College School of Medicine, St Mary's Hospital, London, UK

Anne-Noelle Taquet
Bone and Cartilage Metabolism Unit, Department of Epidemiology and Public Health, University of Liège, Liège, Belgium

Gert-Jan CM van den Bend
Department of Internal Medicine, Erasmus University Medical School, Rotterdam, The Netherlands

Johannes PTM van Leeuwen
Department of Internal Medicine, Erasmus University Medical School, Rotterdam, The Netherlands

Karen Walker-Bone
Medical Research Council Environmental Epidemiology Unit, University of Southampton, Southampton General Hospital, Southampton, UK

Preface

Selective oestrogen receptor modulators represent one of the most exciting therapeutic discoveries of the past decade. Recognition of the potential for compounds to exhibit tissue-specificity and hence avoid unwanted oestrogenic effects has stimulated the development of a number of SERMs with the aim of producing the ideal pharmacological profile. The rapid advances which have recently been made in our understanding of oestrogen signalling pathways have provided some clarification, albeit incomplete, of the mechanisms by which tissue specificity may be achieved and should facilitate the development of better SERMs in the future.

This book provides an up-to-date overview of the pharmacological and clinical profile of SERMs and discusses their potential in maintaining health in the postmenopause. The mechanisms by which SERMs may act are discussed in the light of new discoveries about oestrogen receptors and signalling and the effects of SERMs in the many oestrogen-responsive tissues are addressed in some detail. The role of raloxifene in the management of postmenopausal osteoporosis is reviewed and there is comprehensive coverage of the applications, both realised and potential, of SERMs in the treatment and prevention of breast cancer. SERMs already have an established role in clinical practice in the management of breast cancer and postmenopausal osteoporosis: the challenge for the future will be to extend their use to other major diseases of the postmenopause.

1

Oestrogen deficiency: an overview

Fergus SJ Keating, Nikolay Manassiev, John C Stevenson

Oestrogen deficiency is a potentially deleterious state in postmenopausal women, with multiple effects upon various organ systems that can lead to increased risk of disease. With an increasing ageing population in the developed world, this could represent an enormous burden upon the health systems of countries and it is therefore desirable to identify the manifestations of oestrogen deficiency and to offer treatment to prevent or reverse these effects if possible.

Introduction

Increasingly it is recognized that oestrogen deficiency should be regarded as a gender specific pathological state. The majority of research into oestrogen deficiency has centred on studies of menopausal women. The menopause has been defined by the World Health Organization (WHO) as the permanent cessation of menstruation resulting from the loss of ovarian follicular activity,[1] and the mean age of menopause in the Western world is 51–53 years.[2] The menopause is by its nature a retrospectively diagnosed, discrete event, and by convention is confirmed after 1 year of amenorrhoea, although symptoms reflective of declining ovarian activity commonly commence up to 5 years before the menopause occurs.

Life expectancy in the developed world has increased steadily during the twentieth century, and women commonly live more than one-third of their life in a postmenopausal state. In the UK, 20% of the entire population comprises women over 45 years of age and this represents about 10 million women in an oestrogen deficient state.[3] The potential ramifications of these statistics upon health services have recently begun to be more fully understood as greater knowledge of the effects of oestrogen deficiency on the various organ systems have been elucidated. As discussed below, oestrogen deficiency has been linked to osteoporosis and coronary heart disease (CHD). The financial impact of osteoporosis alone has been estimated to amount to £800 million in the UK[4] with some 60 000 hip fractures each year, leading to 40 premature deaths every day.[5] CHD is the leading cause of death in women in the UK and USA, with 25% of deaths in women attributable to ischaemic heart disease.[6] CHD presents an enormous financial burden to the economies of the developed world, currently estimated at £10 billion per year in the UK alone (total including both direct and indirect costs to the economy).[7] The effects of oestrogen deficiency are thus important to establish and prevent if possible. This chapter will present an overview of the current understanding of oestrogen deficiency on various target organs, but first it is necessary to summarize the structure and mechanism of action of oestrogens.

Oestrogens

Oestrogen describes a group of steroid hormones produced primarily in the ovaries during their reproductive life, but additionally in extra-gonadal sites such as adipose tissue. The ovary produces oestradiol and oestrone (and oestriol) (***Figure 1***). Oestradiol is the primary oestrogen during reproductive life, secreted by the granulosa cells of the developing follicle in response to follicle stimulating hormone (FSH) and lutinizing hormone (LH) secretion from the anterior pituitary gland (***Figure 2***). Oestradiol concentration varies throughout the menstrual cycle, with low levels in the early follicular phase (150–200 pmol/l), a peak at mid-cycle (1200–2600 pmol/l) and intermediate levels (700 pmol/l) in the luteal phase. A small amount of oestrone is also produced, derived mainly by peripheral conversion of androstenedione in adipose tissue, but the ratio of oestradiol to oestrone in the premenopausal woman remains at around 3:1. The daily production of oestradiol during the reproductive years is between 0.07 and 0.8 mg/day, dependent upon the phase of the cycle.[8] Endogenous oestrogens are primarily

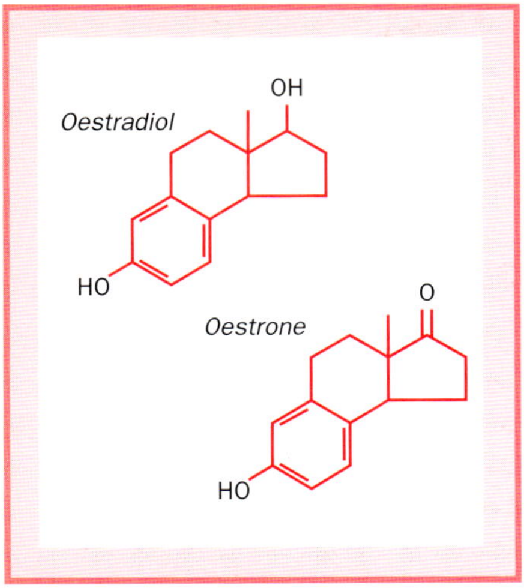

Figure 1
Chemical structure of oestradiol and oestrone.

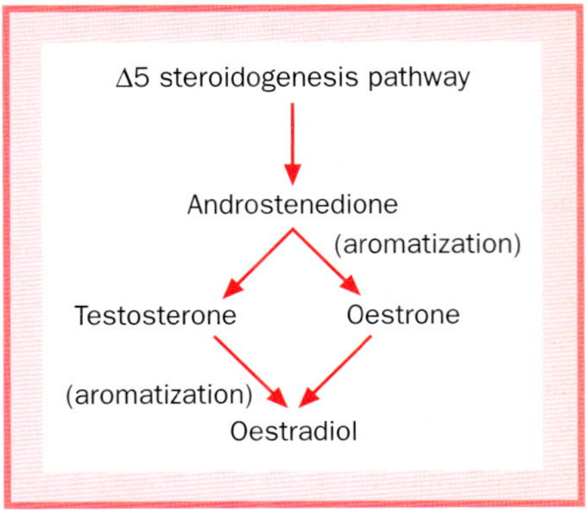

Figure 2
Production of oestradiol and oestrone in the ovary from steroid intermediates.

metabolized in the liver, where they are conjugated with glucuronide (and sulphate) to form water-soluble products, and then excreted in the bile and urine in an inactive form.

In the years leading to the menopause, the numbers of remaining follicles decline, and appear to be more resistant to FSH stimulation. Remaining follicles mature irregularly, with frequent anovulatory cycles and subsequent variable oestrogen secretion; but overall, the level of oestrogen declines. Negative feedback upon FSH production therefore decreases and FSH levels increase, reaching a peak at the menopause. Following the menopause, oestradiol levels are commonly below 110 pmol/l, but the peripheral conversion of androstenedione to oestrone increases. Postmenopause, oestradiol levels decrease by 90% and oestrone levels by 66%, leading to a reversal of the oestradiol:oestrone ratio to 1:3.[9] Oestrone becomes the primary oestrogen of the postmenopause, but the potency of this oestrogen is only 8.5% compared with oestradiol. Consequently, the classical symptoms of oestrogen deficiency develop, as discussed below.

Mechanism of action of oestrogens

Free steroids are thought to diffuse passively to all cells and as yet there is no evidence of an active transport mechanism. Steroids are preferentially retained in target cells as stable complexes with intracellular receptor proteins (i.e. oestrogen receptor, ER), which are steroid and tissue specific. The receptor is thought to be a ligand-activated transcription factor, the steroid being the ligand. The ER has six structural domains of overlapping functions labelled A to F. Two important domains are the steroid-binding domain and the DNA-binding domain. Steroid binding to the receptor results in conformational changes in the hormone-receptor complex, including its DNA-binding domain. This activation process allows the hormone-receptor complex to bind to specific sites on the DNA, termed nuclear acceptor sites. Once bound to the nuclear acceptor sites, the activated steroid-receptor complex acts as a transcription factor, which 'switches on' genes. Specific genes become activated by this process to produce new proteins, which change the metabolism of the target cell in a specific manner. The transfer of the steroid in the cell and nuclear binding of the steroid-receptor complex is rapid, occurring within minutes. Nuclear binding affects mRNA levels and synthesis within several hours, and finally protein synthesis and turnover occurs within 12–24 hours. The major physiological effects of steroids in cells are seen in 12–36 hours.[10]

Symptoms of oestrogen deficiency

Oestrogen deficiency symptoms commonly first manifest during the perimenopause when ovarian function begins to diminish. The most usual oestrogen deficiency symptoms during this time are vasomotor symptoms, psychological symptoms and atrophic changes in oestrogen-sensitive tissues.

Vasomotor symptoms include hot flushes, night sweats, palpitations, headaches and dizziness. Some 80% or more of women will suffer from hot flushes, which are believed to be a manifestation of hypothalamic thermoregulatory dysfunction. Hypo-oestrogenism per se does not strictly cause hot flushes because these are often absent in established postmenopausal women and premenopausal hypo-oestrogenic states such as anorexia nervosa and hyperprolactinaemia. Instead, it is felt that declining levels of oestrogen are responsible for the onset of symptoms.

Psychological symptoms account for a high degree of postmenopausal morbidity, with one study reporting that 86% of women attending a menopause clinic were suffering from a significant psychological morbidity.[11] The commonest symptoms include depression, irritability, tiredness and loss of libido. Oestrogen deficiency is undoubtedly only one of several possible aetiological factors responsible for the prevalence of these symptoms in peri- and postmenopausal women.

Atrophic changes resulting from oestrogen deficiency in sensitive tissues affect the urogenital tract and more generally the skin, hair and nails. Genital tract changes result in atrophic vaginitis, leading to vaginal soreness and dyspareunia. Cervical atrophy and uterine body and endometrial atrophy occur. Urinary tract changes are discussed later. The skin generally thins and loses elasticity and nails become brittle. The underlying mechanisms of these changes will be discussed below.

Oestrogen deficiency and the cardiovascular system

Oestrogen receptors have been demonstrated in canine peripheral and coronary arteries, in cultured rat aortic smooth muscle cells, in baboon myocardium and aorta, and in human endothelial cells.[12,13] Vasodilatation in response to oestrogen administration was first noted in the rabbit ear artery and later in primate coronary arteries, and human umbilical and coronary arteries.[14] It appears that the effect of oestrogen on the cardiovascular system is complex, acting via at least seven different mechanisms, as outlined in *Table 1*.[15]

Table 1
Effects of oestrogen on the CVS.

- *Beneficial effect on blood lipids and lipoproteins*
- *Positive effect on endothelial cell function*
- *Relaxation of the vascular smooth muscle*
- *Decreases platelet adhesion and aggregation*
- *Effects on coagulation and fibrinolysis*
- *Promotes and maintains gynaecoid body fat distribution*
- *Improves glucose and insulin metabolism*

Effect of oestrogen deficiency on vasculature

The response of vessels to oestrogen is largely vasodilatory. Under the influence of oestrogen, cardiac output increases, systemic vascular resistance decreases, and blood pressure remains unchanged. In the cerebrovascular circulation, there are gender differences. Before the menopause, cerebrovascular blood flow is greater in women than in men of the same age. Cerebrovascular blood flow is increased in pregnancy, when oestrogen levels are also increased, but decreases after the menopause. Oestrogen affects the reactivity of cerebral arteries to vasoactive stimuli such as serotonin.[14]

As yet, the mechanism of oestrogen's effects on the vasculature has not been fully elucidated, but several explanations have been proposed, involving either immediate or delayed effects. Immediate effects are likely to result from nitric oxide (NO) production and prostaglandin formation from the endothelium and effects of calcium channels in the smooth muscle cells on the vessel wall. Longer-lasting effects may involve reducing angiotensin-converting enzyme activity,[16] inhibition of smooth muscle cell proliferation and increasing the smooth muscle cell prostaglandin production by increasing prostacyclin synthetase and cyclo-oxygenase.[17]

The normal effect of endogenous oestrogen in premenopausal women, as described above, is found in postmenopausal women given physiological doses of oestrogen. Both endothelium-dependent and endothelium-independent blood flow improves in the coronary and brachial arteries of postmenopausal women with CHD in response to oestrogen.[14,17] In the cerebrovascular circulation, the pulsatility index (PI), as measured with Doppler ultrasound in the region of the internal carotid artery, increases following menopause.[18] PI is thought to represent the impedance to blood flow distal to the probe: the higher the impedance, the higher the PI. Oestrogen also reverses the paradoxical constriction of diseased coronary arteries by acetylcholine.[19]

Effect of oestrogen deficiency on lipids and lipoprotein metabolism

Oestrogen deficiency following the menopause is associated with changes in blood lipids and lipoproteins. Studies examining these changes have consistently shown that there is a significant increase in total cholesterol, low density lipoprotein (LDL) cholesterol and triglycerides, and a decrease in high density lipoprotein (HDL) cholesterol after adjustment for age, body mass index and smoking.[19–22] The important HDL2 subfraction was found to be reduced as a direct result of the menopause.[22] Premenopausal women have lower hepatic lipase activity than men of the same age and their HDL is higher. Premenopausal women also have a more favourable lipid profile than men, with their LDL lower until the sixth decade, lower very low density lipoprotein (VLDL) throughout life, and higher HDL during postpubertal life. The differences are due to increased apo B100 receptor activity in the cell membrane, leading to lower LDL, more efficient clearance of VLDL, an increased rate of synthesis and a reduced clearance of HDL. Hepatic lipase activity is higher in men than in women, hence HDL is lower in men. Lipoprotein(a) increases after the age of 50, as does fibrinogen.[23]

Effect of oestrogen deficiency on body fat distribution

Oestrogen promotes and maintains the deposition of adipose tissue in the classic gynaecoid pattern of postpubertal females. Waist-to-hip ratio measurements and dual-energy X-ray absorptiometry (DEXA) measurements show that there is a postmenopausal shift in fat deposition, with a significant increase in abdominal (android) and intra-abdominal fat distribution.[24] This may result from a fall in oestrogen levels and a fall of the oestrogen:androgen ratio after the menopause. This increase in waist-to-hip ratio over time in women has been shown to be associated with a significant increase in cardiovascular morbidity and mortality.[25]

Effect of oestrogen deficiency on glucose and insulin metabolism

Oestrogen deficiency leads to decreased insulin output from the pancreas, decreased insulin elimination and relative insulin resistance.[26] Whilst hyperglycaemia itself may result in injury to the vascular endothelium, it is insulin resistance with accompanying hyperinsulinaemia that may be a pivotal metabolic disturbance in the pathogenesis of CHD.

Effect of oestrogen deficiency on coagulation and fibrinolysis

It has been shown that increased levels of Factor VII and fibrinogen are risk factors for cardiovascular disease.[27] The association of those two factors with cardiovascular death appears to be at least as strong as the association between cholesterol and cardiovascular death. The menopause itself leads to a 6% increase in the level of Factor VII and a 10% increase in fibrinogen.[28,29] Orally administered 17-ßoestradiol seems to decrease the level of fibrinogen.[30] Oestrogen enhances fibrinolysis in postmenopausal women by reducing plasminogen activator inhibitor-1 by 50%.[31] Little is known about the effect of the menopause on platelet function, but it appears that exogenous oestrogen (as hormone replacement therapy, HRT) decreases platelet aggregation and adenosine triphosphate release.[32]

The complex relationship between oestrogen and coagulation is not fully understood, and is complicated by the emerging evidence of a significant positive correlation between exogenous oestrogen administration and venous thromboembolism, whereas endogenous oestrogen deficiency seems to be correlated with arterial thrombosis, and increased risk and incidence of CHD and cerebrovascular disease.[33]

Oestrogen deficiency and the skeleton

As discussed earlier, the development of postmenopausal osteoporosis represents a major public health issue. Osteoporosis has been defined as 'a disease characterised by low bone mass and micro-architectural deterioration of bone tissue, leading to enhanced bone fragility and a consequent increase in fracture risk'.[34] The development of osteoporosis depends upon both the peak bone mass attained and its subsequent rate of loss. Peak bone mass is achieved in early adulthood and is largely genetically determined. This has been confirmed in studies comparing bone mass in twins and in studies of racial groups that have migrated. To some extent, peak bone mass is influenced by diet, exercise, alcohol consumption, smoking, drugs (e.g. corticosteroids, contraceptive pills, liver enzyme inducers), parity and the presence or absence of oestrogens.[35] The rate of bone loss is influenced by factors that affect the balance between bone formation and resorption. Oestrogens seem to have a central role in regulating bone mass, and oestrogen-deficient states such as anorexia nervosa, secondary amenorrhoea due to strenuous exercise, use of gonadotropin inhibitors and menopause have all been shown to lead to bone loss.[36]

The development of osteoporosis results from an imbalance between bone resorption and bone formation. The loss of gonadal function and ageing are the two most important factors. Starting around the fourth or fifth decade of life, men and women lose 0.3–0.5% of their bone mass every year. This is increased in women by up to tenfold after the loss of gonadal function due to an increase in bone turnover, and women may eventually lose up to 50% of their cancellous bone and 30% of their cortical bone. There are indications that, in the early years following surgical or natural menopause, there is a period of accelerated bone loss, which in later life decreases but continues into old age.

Mechanism of action of oestrogen on bone

Oestrogens are thought to affect the bone both directly and indirectly.

Direct actions

Studies on osteoblast-like osteosarcoma cells and in human osteoblast-like cells have shown that these possess oestrogen receptors. Oestrogen binds to the receptors and, through the classical oestrogen receptor mediated mechanism, leads to response from the cells which may include the production of type I collagen and transforming growth factor beta.[37,38]

Oestrogen also acts through locally produced factors: cytokines, growth factors and prostaglandins. Cytokines (IL-1, IL-6), tumour necrosis factors and transforming growth factor-β are potent inducers of bone resorption and osteoclast formation. They are secreted by stromal cells in the bone marrow and by osteoclasts. It has been suggested that oestrogens inhibit IL-6 and perhaps other cytokines. The changes in bone turnover are most pronounced where metabolic activity is high such as in cancellous bone.[39]

Indirect actions

Oestrogens may alter the set point at which parathyroid hormone (PTH) responds to calcium, thus reducing PTH secretion and the rate of bone turnover. It may also stimulate intestinal calcium absorption by enhancing renal 1,25-dihydroxyvitamin D synthesis. It may also enhance secretion of calcitonin, a hormone that inhibits bone resorption.

Oestrogen deficiency and the urogenital system

Embryological development of the primitive urogenital sinus leads to the formation of the female genital and urological tracts, and oestrogen receptors have been isolated in the tissues of the vagina, urethra, bladder and pelvic floor. Prolonged oestrogen deficiency is associated with urological complaints including frequency, nocturia, incontinence, urinary tract infections and the 'urge syndrome', as well as the classic vaginal symptoms of oestrogen deficiency: dryness, itching, burning and dyspareunia.[40]

Although the prevalence of urinary incontinence increases with age, oestrogen deficiency is only one of several causes, and the menopause has not been specifically linked to the onset of incontinence.[41] Incontinence arises when the urethral closure pressure is exceeded by the intravesical pressure. Oestrogen may exert beneficial effects on positive urethral pressure by a combination of increased urethral cell maturation and periurethral collagen production, increased blood flow and increased α-adrenoreceptor sensitivity in the urethral smooth muscle. Oestrogens may also raise the sensory threshold of the bladder and reduce the incidence of urinary tract infection.[40]

Oestrogen deficiency and the skin

The menopause may affect all organs containing connective tissue. Oestrogen and androgen receptors have been found on dermal fibroblasts,[42] and further work has elucidated the presence of receptors in the epidermis, hair follicles, sebaceous glands, eccrine glands and vessels.[43] Postmenopausal atrophy of the dermis results from a decrease in the dermal skin collagen content, and although it is not clear whether the changes are due to the ageing process, it has been shown that oestrogen administration reverses the process.[44]

Skin collagen content declines in the first 5 years after the menopause by up to 30%,[45] and work has shown that skin collagen content and skin thickness are increased in women on HRT compared with age-matched women receiving no treatment.[44] The hypo-oestrogenic state thus has a profound effect on skin which can lead to a rapid loss of structure and function that is preventable and reversible with adequate oestrogen replacement.

Oestrogen deficiency and the CNS

Oestrogen receptors have been demonstrated in the cortex, limbic system, hippocampus, cerebellum, locus ceruleus, hypothalamus, preoptic area and amygdala, and are thus able to modify the synthesis, release and metabolism of neurotransmitters in these areas. Oestrogens are also believed to influence dynamic processes whereby neurites are extended, synaptic connections are formed and neuronal circuits are modelled. Thus, the activity of the hypothalamic thermoregulatory, satiety/appetite and blood pressure areas, and the limbic system regulation of mood tone and psychological well being may be influenced in a global sense by oestrogen.[46] Oestrogen deficiency at these specific sites in the CNS is thought to be responsible therefore for many of the climacteric symptoms reported by women, including hot flushes, sweats and disturbances in mood.

Recent attention has focused on the role of oestrogen deficiency in cognitive function, and the link, if any, between oestrogen deficiency and Alzheimer's disease. Data from epidemiological studies have shown that chronic degenerative diseases of the CNS including Alzheimer's disease and Parkinson's disease are more common in women than in age-matched males. Oestrogens have been demonstrated to increase cholinergic tone, which is positively linked to memory performance.[47,48] The decline in short-term memory following the menopause may be attributable to the effects of oestrogen deficiency on the neurotransmitter acetylcholine. Oestrogen increases levels of acetyltransferase, the enzyme involved in acetylcholine synthesis,[49] and thus oestrogen deficiency may lead to reductions of this critical transmitter involved in many cognitive processes such as attention processing, learning and memory. Oestrogen deficiency may lead to decreased cerebral blood flow as discussed above. Postmenopausal oestrogen deprivation has thus been postulated as a risk factor for Alzheimer's disease, and oestrogen replacement given to Alzheimer's patients has been shown to improve measures of cognitive performance.[50] However, evidence for an absolute cause and effect relationship between oestrogen deficiency and Alzheimer's disease is as yet inconclusive. Further work will hopefully establish the precise nature of any relationship.

Conclusion

It can therefore be seen that oestrogen deficiency produces major alterations in the functioning of many of the female organ systems, and that these changes can be potentially detrimental and disease provoking. Traditionally, the menopause has been viewed as an inevitable consequence of ageing, and oestrogen deficiency accepted as a natural consequence of this process. However, this review of the effects of oestrogen deficiency has shown that replacement of oestrogen, which traditionally has been accomplished by the use of oestrogen in HRT, but more recently potentially achieved with the use of novel selective oestrogen receptor modulators (SERMs), may have an enormous impact in the quality of life and the prevention of disease in postmenopausal women.

References

1. World Health Organization. Research on the menopause in the 1990s. Reports of a WHO scientific group. WHO: Geneva, 1996.
2. McKinley SM, Brambilla DJ, Posner JG. The normal menopause transition. *Am J Hum Biol* 1992; **4**: 37–46.
3. Office of Population Censuses and Surveys. Mortality statistics cause 1990, Series DH2, No. 17. HMSO: London, 1991.
4. Smith R, Studd JWW. *The Menopause and Hormone Replacement Therapy.* Martin Dunitz, London, 1993: 10–11.
5. Cummings SR, Kesley JL, Nevitt MC et al. Epidemiology of osteoporosis and osteoporotic fractures. *Epidemiol Rev* 1995; **7**: 178–208.
6. Marmot MG, Mann JI. Ischaemic heart disease. Epidemiology and prevention. In: Weatherall DJ, Ledingham JGG, Warrel DA (eds). *Oxford Textbook of Medicine.* Oxford University Press: Oxford, 1996: 2305–18.
7. Maniadakis N. Coronary heart disease statistics: economic cost supplement. British Heart Foundation: London, 1999 (in press).
8. Carr BR. The ovary. In: Carr BR, Blackwell RE (eds). *Textbook of Reproductive Medicine.* Appleton & Lange: Norwalk, USA. 1993: 199–200.
9. Watson N. Pathophysiology of the menopause In: Ress M (ed). *Menopause. Update Postgraduate Centre Series.* Reed Healthcare Communications: Sutton, Surrey, UK. 1995: 9–11.
10. Speroff L, Glass RH, Kase NG. Hormone biosynthesis, metabolism and mechanism of action. In: Speroff L, Glass RH, Kase NG (eds). *Clinical Gynecological Endocrinology and Infertility.* Williams and Wilkins: Baltimore MD, USA. 1978: 19.
11. Montgomery JC, Studd JWW. Psychological and sexual aspects of the menopause. *Br J Hosp Med* 1991; **34**: 300–2.
12. Lin AL, Gonzalez R, Carey K, Shain SA. Estradiol 17-beta affects estrogen receptor distribution and elevates progesterone receptor content in baboon aorta. *Atherosclerosis* 1986; **6**: 495–504.
13. Lordoso DW, Kearney M, Kim EA, Jekanowski J, Isner JM. Variable expression of estrogen receptor in normal and atherosclerotic coronary arteries of premenopausal women. *Circulation* 1994; **89**: 1501–10.
14. Collins P. Vascular aspects of oestrogen. *Maturitas* 1996; **23**: 217–26.
15. Stevenson JC. Mechanisms whereby oestrogens influence arterial health. *Eur J Obstet Gynaecol* 1996; **65**: 39–42.
16. Proudler AJ, Ahmed HAI, Crook D, Fogelman I, Rymer J, Stevenson JC. Hormone replacement therapy and serum angiotensin converting enzyme activity in postmenopausal women. *Lancet* 1995; **346**: 89–90.
17. Mendelsohn ME, Karas RH. Oestrogen and the blood vessel wall. *Curr Opin Cardiol* 1994; **9**: 619–26.
18. Gangar KF, Vyas S, Whitehead M, Crook D, Miere H, Campbell S. Pulsatility index in the internal carotid artery in relation to transdermal oestradiol and time since menopause. *Lancet* 1991; **338**: 834–42.

19. Collins P, Rosano GMC, Sarrel PM et al. 17β-estradiol attenuates acetylcholine-induced coronary arterial constriction in women but not men with coronary heart disease. *Circulation* 1995; **92**: 24–30.

20. Bonithon-Copp C, Scarabin PY, Darne B et al. Menopause related changes in lipoproteins and some other cardiovascular risk factors. *Int J Epidemiol* 1990; **19**: 42–8.

21. Jensen J, Nilas L, Christiansen C. Influence of menopause on serum lipids and lipoproteins. *Maturitas* 1990; **12**: 321–31.

22. Stevenson J, Crook D, Godsland I. Effects of age and menopause on lipid metabolism of healthy women. *Atherosclerosis* 1993; **98**: 83–90.

23. Assmann G, Cullen P, Schulte H. HRT, plasma risk factors and cardiovascular disease. *Eur Menopause J* 1996; **3**: 203–8.

24. Ley CJ, Lees B, Stevenson JC. Sex and menopause associated changes in body fat distribution. *Am J Clin Nutr* 1992; **55**: 950–4.

25. Lapidus L, Bengtsson C, Larsson B, Pennert K, Rybo T, Sjostrom L. Distribution of adipose tissue and risk of cardiovascular disease and death: a 12 year follow up of participants in the population study of Gothenburg, Sweden. *Br Med J* 1984; **289**: 1257–61.

26. Gaspard UJ, Gottal J-M, den Brule FA. Postmenopausal changes of lipid and glucose metabolism: a review of their main aspects. *Maturitas* 1995; **21**: 171–8.

27. Meade TW, North WRS, Chakrabarti R, Sterling Y, Haines AP, Thompson SG. Haemostatic function and cardiovascular death: early results of a prospective study. *Lancet* 1980; **i**: 1050–4.

28. Meade TW, Haines AP, Imerson JD, Sterling Y. Thompson SG. Menopausal status and haemostatic variables. *Lancet* 1983; **i**: 22–4.

29. Meade TW, Ruddock V, Sterling Y, Chakrabarti R, Miller JG. Fibrinolytic activity, clotting factors and long-term incidence of ischaemic heart disease in the Northwick Park heart study. *Lancet* 1993; **342**: 1076–9.

30. Gilbert J, Estelles A, Cano A et al. The effect of estrogen replacement therapy with or without progestogen on the fibrinolytic system and coagulation inhibitors in postmenopausal women. *Am J Obstet Gynecol* 1995; **793**: 1849–54.

31. Koh KK, Mincemoyer R, Bui MN et al. Effects of hormone replacement therapy on fibrinolysis in postmenopausal women. *N Engl J Med* 1997; **336**: 683–90.

32. Bar J, Tepper R, Fuchs J et al. The effect of estrogen replacement therapy on platelet aggregation and adenosine triphosphate release in postmenopausal women. *Obstet Gynecol* 1993; **81**: 261–4.

33. Lowe G. Effects of oestrogen on thromboembolism. In: Sturdee D (ed). *HRT and Thromboembolism.* Royal Society of Medicine Press: London, 1997: 3–4.

34. Anonymous Consensus Development Conference 1991. Prophylaxis and treatment of osteoporosis. *Am J Med* 1991; **90**: 107–10.

35. Ralston SH. Osteoporosis. *BMJ* 1997; **315**: 469–72.

36. Rizzoli R, Bonjour J-P. Hormones and bones. *Lancet* 1997; **349**: S20–3.

37. Komm BS, Terpening CM, Benz DJ et al. Estrogen binding, receptor mRNA, and biologic response in osteoblast-like osteosarcoma cells. *Science* 1988; **241**: 81–3.

38. Eriksen EF, Colvard DS, Berg NJ et al. Evidence of oestrogen receptors in normal human osteoblast-like cells. *Science* 1988; **241**: 84–6.

39. Manolagas SC, Jilka RL. Bone marrow, cytokines, and bone remodeling. *N Engl J Med* 1995; **332**: 305–11.

40. Hextall A, Cardozo L. The effect of estrogen deficiency on the bladder. In: Studd JW (ed). *The Management of the Menopause. Annual Review 1998.* Parthenon Publishing Group: Carnforth, UK, 1998: 39–45.

41. Thomas TM, Plymat KR, Blannin J, Meade TW. Prevalence of urinary incontinence. *Br Med J* 1980; **281**: 1243–5.

42. Stumpf WE, Sar M, Joshi SG. Estrogen target cells in the skin. *Experientia* 1974; **30**: 196–8.

43. Jemec GB, Wojnarowska F. The distribution of p29 protein in normal human skin. *Br J Dermatol* 1987; **117**: 217–24.

44. Brincat MP, Galea R. Estrogens and skin. In: Studd JW (ed). *The Management of the Menopause. Annual Review 1998.* Parthenon Publishing Group: Carnforth, UK, 1998: 19–25.

45. Brincat M, Moniz CF, Studd JWW et al. Sex hormones and skin collagen content in postmenopausal women. *Br Med J* 1983; **287**: 1337–8.

46. Genazzani AR, Salvestroni C, Spinetti A, Montelone P, Petraglia F. Estrogens and neurotransmitters. In: Studd JW (ed). *The Management of the Menopause. Annual Review 1998.* Parthenon Publishing Group: Carnforth, UK, 1998: 169–75.

47. Luine VN. Estradiol increases choline acetyltransferase activity in specific basal forebrain nuclei and projection areas of female rats. *Exp Neurol* 1985; **80**: 484–90.

48. Bartus RT, Dean RL, Beer B et al. The cholinergic hypothesis of geriatric memory dysfunction. *Science* 1981; **217**: 208–17.

49. Philips S, Sherwin BB. Effects of estrogen on memory function in surgically menopausal women. *Psychoneuroendocrinology* 1992; **17**: 485–95.

50. Henderson VW. Estrogens and prevention of Alzheimer's disease. In: Studd JW (ed). *The Management of the Menopause. Annual Review 1998.* Parthenon Publishing Group: Carnforth, UK, 1998: 183–9.

2

Epidemiology of the menopause

Karen Walker-Bone, Cyrus Cooper

Oestrogen deficiency after the menopause has important public health associations with chronic disease (ischaemic heart disease and osteoporosis). The role of HRT in the prevention of these diseases is yet to be elucidated.

Introduction

The menopause has assumed far greater importance since the beginning of this century due to dramatic shifts in the age structures of Western populations. Historical data show that the average lifespan of men and women in Roman times was 25 years. In Elizabethan England, the average female life expectancy was 40 years and only 25% of women lived long enough to experience the menopause. However, during the last century, there have been dramatic reductions in infant, child and maternal mortality, leading to a rapid increase in the life expectancy of women.[1] Currently, average female life expectancy is approaching 80 years (***Figure 2.1***).

Despite these demographic changes, the average age at menopause has changed little throughout the centuries and

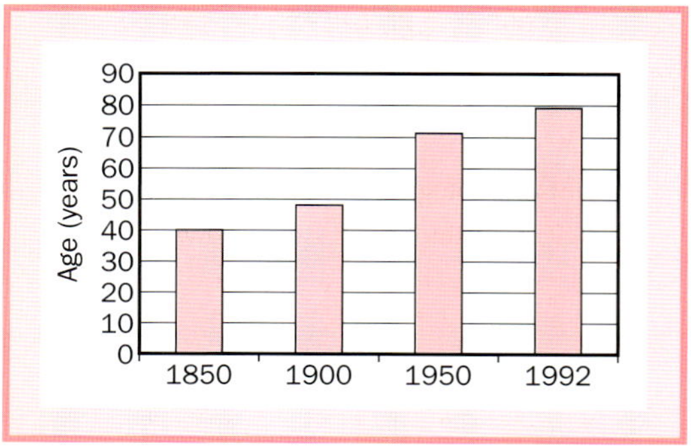

Figure 2.1
Life expectancy of women at birth. Data adapted from ref. 2.

remains consistently around 51 years. Therefore, approximately 95% of women born today live to experience the menopause and the average woman now lives 30 years (or 40% of her adult life) after the menopause.[3] Furthermore, it is predicted that these demographic shifts will continue. For example, in the United Kingdom, there are currently almost 10 million women aged over 50 years, who make up 17% of the total United Kingdom population. It has been estimated that by the year 2029 there will be 12.5 million women aged over 50 years, who will comprise 20% of the total population.

The term *menopause* literally signifies the permanent cessation of menstruation due to loss of ovarian follicular function. In clinical practice, it is diagnosed retrospectively after 12 months of amenorrhoea. The menopause is a discrete physiological event, which will be experienced by every woman who lives beyond the age of 60 years. However, there is a transition phase leading up to the menopause which may take from 2 to 8 years, during which there is a gradual reduction in ovarian follicular activity. This phase is referred to as the *perimenopause* (or *climacteric*) and may manifest clinically as menstrual irregularity accompanied by postmenopausal symptoms of oestrogen deficiency.

Knowledge of the menopause and its consequences has broadened rapidly, by necessity, over the last 20–30 years. With so many women living after the menopause, the most important public health consequence is the association between oestrogen deficiency and chronic disease (osteoporosis and ischaemic heart disease). These are the major causes of morbidity and mortality in ageing women and the role of oestrogen deficiency in their development is particularly important because of the potential for prevention with hormone replacement therapy (HRT). However, HRT is a complex intervention that may have beneficial and adverse specific health effects, and this review will address both of these.

Demography of the menopause

Age at menarche and at menopause: the number of fertile years

The mean age at menarche among girls in the Western world is gradually decreasing, with data from Europe showing that the current mean age is 13.7 years.[4] This gradual reduction has been attributed to improvements in health and living conditions. Remarkably, however, age at menopause has remained consistent over centuries. Since records began in the sixth century, the average age at menopause has remained at about 50 years; moreover, worldwide estimates fall consistently within the range 49–51 years.[5] Therefore, the average number of fertile years experienced by women is gradually increasing simply as a result of the younger age at menarche.

Factors that influence age at menopause

Cigarette smoking

Epidemiological studies have shown that cigarette smoking is associated with a significant reduction in age at menopause, such that women who currently smoke experience the menopause an average of 1.5 years before non-smokers.[6] There is a dose–response relationship whereby the number of cigarettes smoked and the duration of smoking correlate with an earlier age at menopause. Furthermore, ever-smokers experience the menopause earlier than never-smokers. The mechanism of association between smoking and age at menopause has not been clarified, although it has been postulated that cigarette smoke induces a more rapid metabolism of exogenous oestrogen, or that components of cigarette smoke, such as aromatic hydrocarbons, might speed up the rate at which oocytes mature.

Nutritional status

Research in Papua New Guinea has shown that malnourished women experience the menopause an average of 4 years earlier than those who are well-nourished.[5] It has been hypothesized that the mechanism for this effect might be the influence of nutritional status on body build. Malnutrition is associated with lower height and weight, both of which may have an influence on age at menopause.

Gynaecological surgery

The menopause occurs earlier in women who have had a total abdominal hysterectomy.[7] It is thought that the operation might compromise the ovarian blood supply, thereby precipitating earlier oocyte insufficiency.

Altitude

A consistent association has been discovered with altitude, such that women living at high altitude experience the menopause earlier.

Other risk factors

Possible associations have been investigated with other factors, such as racial origin, age at menarche, parity, use of oral contraceptives, socio-economic history, and maternal age at menopause, but no consistent associations have been found. Cigarette smoking may well be a confounder for some of these variables.[5]

Manifestations of the menopause

These can best be divided into two groups: acute symptoms at the time of the menopause and chronic syndromes as a result of long-term oestrogen deficiency. Hormone replacement therapy has a role in the relief of the acute perimenopausal symptoms and in the prevention, or treatment, of chronic diseases.

Acute postmenopausal symptoms

Vasomotor symptoms

It is thought that the most characteristic symptoms of the perimenopausal period are caused by vasomotor instability: hot flushes, night sweats, palpitations and headaches.[8] These symptoms are experienced by approximately 75% of perimenopausal women in Western societies, although it is not certain why 25% of women do not experience such symptoms. There are cultural differences in the reporting of these symptoms with as few as 10–20% complaining of symptoms in East Asian societies. This may reflect differences in cultural attitudes towards sexuality, so those women who regard the menopause as part of the normal life cycle are less likely to report perimenopausal symptoms. In all women, these symptoms reduce spontaneously as time from the menopause increases, although it is reported that these symptoms persist indefinitely in 5–10% of women. Treatment with oestrogen is effective in relieving these symptoms in most women. Although a direct link between vasomotor symptoms and the later sequelae of oestrogen deficiency has not been firmly established, evidence is beginning to accrue that women who suffer severe postmenopausal flushing have lower bone mineral density.

Atrophic epithelial changes

Oestrogen deficiency is associated with thinning of the vaginal wall and distal urethra. This leads to vaginal dryness and itching, dyspareunia, urinary frequency and urinary incontinence. Intravaginal oestrogen prevents and treats some of these symptoms, and possibly also reduces the risk of recurrent urinary tract infections. However, urinary incontinence becomes more common with increasing age, and a recent meta-analysis concluded that oestrogens do not effectively treat the symptoms of stress or urge incontinence.[9]

Depression

Affective disorders are more common at the time of the menopause, with as many as 25–50% of women experiencing some type of psychological disturbance; however, there is insufficient evidence that it is the hormonal changes of the menopause which cause depression. There are significant psychosocial stresses associated with this phase of a woman's life, such as coping with loss of fertility, caring for aged parents and children leaving home. It seems likely that these psychosocial stresses, coupled with sleep disturbance caused by vasomotor symptoms, account for the increased prevalence of depression. Research in this area has been hampered by methodological and statistical problems, as well as the temporal problem that menopause is diagnosed retrospectively.[10]

Reduced sexual function

Ageing, and to some extent the perimenopausal symptoms of vaginal atrophy and sleep disturbance, may result in physical symptoms that decrease the opportunities for, and enjoyment of, sexual intimacy. However, there is no evidence that the importance of sexuality decreases in women after the menopause. There is a reduction in the prevalence of sexual activity between the ages of 45 and 64 years, but this might be part of a trend towards declining frequency of sexual activity related to age.

Chronic disease associated with the menopause

Osteoporosis

Osteoporosis is defined as 'a systemic skeletal disease characterized by low bone mass and micro-architectural deterioration of bone tissue leading to enhanced bone fragility and increased propensity to fracture'.[11] The disease is a major health problem because of its causal association with fractures, which typically occur at the hip, distal forearm or spine. The burden of osteoporotic fractures throughout Europe is summarized in ***Table 2.1***.

Osteoporosis is rare in women aged less than 50 years. However, the numbers of women with osteoporosis increase steadily with age. In the USA, less than 15% of women between 50 and 59 years have

Table 2.1
Impact of osteoporosis-related fractures in Europe.

	Hip	Spine	Wrist
Lifetime risk (%)			
women	14	11	13
men	3	2	2
Cases per year	400 000	270 000	330 000
Hospitalization (%)	100	2–10	22
Relative survival	0.83	0.82	1.00

Costs: all sites combined, approximately £10 billion.
Data from ref. 12.

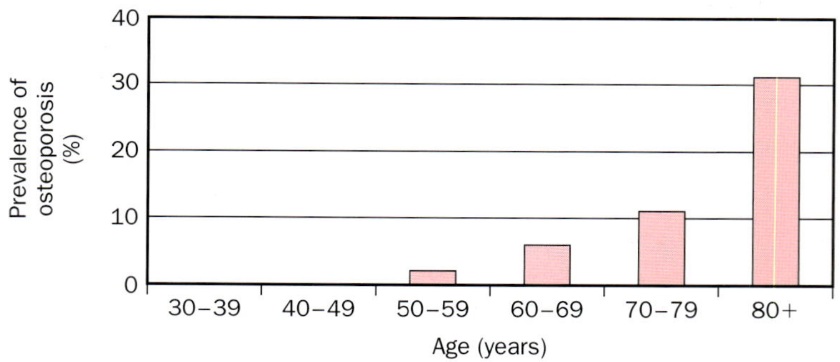

Figure 2.2
Age-stratified prevalence of osteoporosis.

osteoporosis, but by the age of 80 years, 27% are osteopenic and 70% are osteoporotic at either the hip, lumbar spine or distal forearm.[13] Of the osteoporotic group, 60% will have already experienced one or more fragility fractures. By extrapolation, it is estimated that 16.8 million (54%) postmenopausal Caucasian women are osteopenic and a further 9.4 million (30%) are osteoporotic.[14] *Figure 2.2* shows the prevalence of osteoporosis among UK women aged 50 years and above. The prevalence rises from 2% at ages 50–59 years to 31.2% at age 80 years.[15]

Hip fracture

These are the most severe of all the osteoporotic fractures, especially in the elderly.[16] The mortality rate 1 year following hip fracture in women is 21%, with most of the excess deaths occurring within the first 6 months. Of those who survive, mobility remains permanently impaired in over half. In financial terms, hip fractures are a large burden on the healthcare budget. Taking into account inpatient costs, institutional care and rehabilitation, the costs approach £500 million per annum in England.

The risk of hip fracture rises with age, influenced by increases in both the severity of osteoporosis and the frequency of falls. In the UK, the average age at the time of a hip fracture is 79 years. In all, 90% of hip fractures occur among people aged over 50 years and incidence is approximately twice as great in women as in men at all ages above 45 years. This sex difference, coupled with the larger number of women in the elderly population, results in 80% of all cases of hip fracture occurring in women.[17]

There are methodological problems in comparing rates of hip fracture among different races and ethnic groups, but some patterns have emerged. Caucasian populations have higher incidence rates than black populations in North America and South Africa. Furthermore, the female preponderance seen in Caucasians is not found in the other ethnic groups. This may be partly explained by the finding that black people have relatively higher peak bone mass and slower rates of bone turnover. There is marked geographic variation in hip fracture incidence rates throughout Europe (*Figure 2.3*), with the highest rates observed in Scandinavia and the lowest rates in Mediterranean countries. These differences are compatible with an important influence of hypovitaminosis D.

Hip fractures show seasonal variation in incidence, with more fractures occurring in winter than in summer months. However, most hip fractures occur after falls indoors, and are not the result of slipping on icy pavements, suggesting that the winter peak reflects factors such as abnormal neuromuscular function related to lower temperatures, or again, a winter-time reduction in exposure to sunlight and vitamin D insufficiency.

Vertebral fractures

The epidemiology of vertebral fractures has been the most difficult to characterize because of a lack of universally accepted diagnostic criteria and the high proportion of vertebral deformities

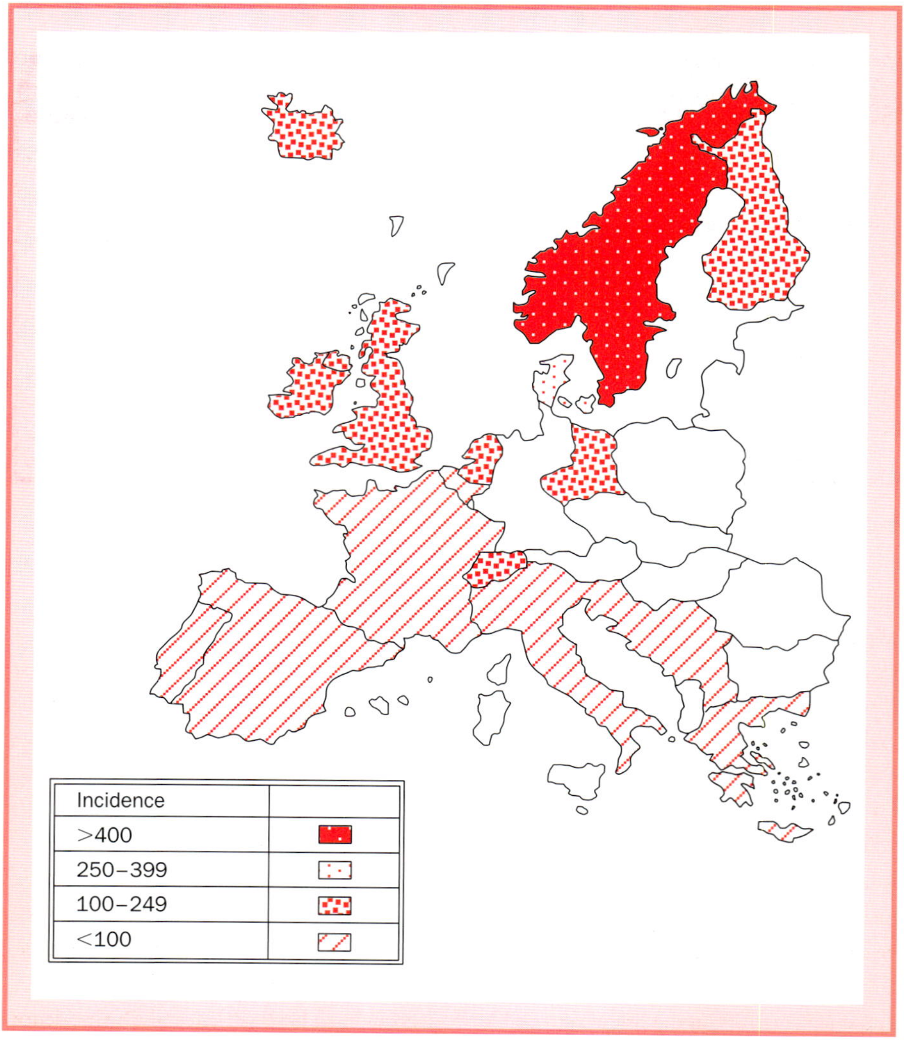

Figure 2.3
Incidence of hip fracture in women in Europe (incidence refers to the crude rate per 100 000 of the population aged 50 years or over). Reproduced with permission from Martin Dunitz Ltd: Meunier (ed) Osteoporosis: Diagnosis and Management, *1998.*

Table 2.2
Hormonal/reproductive variables and risk of vertebral deformity.

Variable		Odds ratio	(95% CI)
Age at menarche (years):	<12	1.0	–
	>16	1.5	(1.2–1.9)
Age at menopause (years):	<45	1.0	–
	>53	0.8	(0.6–1.0)
Use of HRT:	Never	1.0	–
	≥1 year	0.8	(0.6–1.1)
Use of OCP:	Never	1.0	–
	Ever	0.8	(0.6–1.0)

Data from ref. 4.
CI, confidence interval; HRT, hormone replacement therapy; OCP, oral contraceptive pill.

which are subclinical. Early definitions relied on subjective evaluation of radiography and had rather poor reproducibility. Newer techniques rely on vertebral morphometry and have produced more reliable data.

It is estimated that one in eight postmenopausal white women in Europe has radiological evidence of at least one vertebral deformity.[18] Prevalence rates are closer among men and women than for hip fractures, but are consistently greater in women over the age of 65 years. The effects of hormonal and reproductive factors on the risk of vertebral deformity were recently investigated as part of the European Vertebral Osteoporosis Study.[4] Hormonal status was found to be important in the development of vertebral osteoporosis and fractures, such that those in the highest fifth of age at menarche (age > 16 years) had an increased risk of vertebral deformity, whilst lower rates were found among users of HRT and the oral contraceptive and those who were older at the menopause (*Table 2.2*).

The most severe grades of radiological deformity are associated with the following clinical symptoms: back pain, kyphosis, loss of height and disability involving the back. It is common for vertebral fractures to be multiple and this causes cumulative disability, depression and low self-esteem. The incidence of clinically diagnosed vertebral fractures is probably less than one-third of the true incidence, and only 2–8% of incident vertebral fractures lead to hospital admission.

Wrist fractures

Wrist fractures have a different incidence pattern to the other fragility fractures. There is a marked female preponderance, with an age-adjusted ratio of 4:1, so that 80% of these fractures occur in women. However, the age-specific rates show a linear increase from 40 to 65 years and then a plateau. The plateau effect has not been explained, although it is hypothesized that it may reflect perimenopausal changes in trabecular bone content, or a variation in the pattern of falls with age. Wrist fractures are also seasonal, with peaks in winter, particularly in times of freezing weather when falls onto the outstretched hand are frequent. Worldwide studies have suggested that there are ethnic differences in rates.

Wrist fractures do not lead to increased mortality, but they do cause significant morbidity. Only 50% of patients report good functional recovery at 6 months.[19] There are several long-term complications: reflex sympathetic dystrophy, neuropathies and post-traumatic arthritis.

HRT and osteoporosis

Several studies have shown that HRT has a protective effect against postmenopausal bone loss through a reduction in bone turnover,[20] but there is less evidence that HRT reduces the risk of fracture (especially hip fracture) in the elderly.[21] Further, the positive effects of HRT may be lost 5–10 years after discontinuing therapy.[22] Therefore, whilst HRT might be effective as a prophylaxis against fractures in elderly women, it may have to be taken indefinitely. As we will discuss, there are other implications if HRT is taken in the long term.

Ischaemic heart disease

Ischaemic heart disease (IHD) is the most common cause of death in women over the age of 50 years in Western societies. Approximately twice as many women die from IHD as from malignancy. The rates of IHD in premenopausal women are relatively low compared to men. However, the incidence rates gradually rise in the 6–10 years after the menopause (the menopause is associated with an approximate doubling in risk) until they become almost equivalent to those in men.

Risk factors for IHD

There is a triad of potentially modifiable risk factors for IHD: cigarette smoking, hypertension and elevated blood lipids.[23] Cigarette smoking is associated with almost a doubling of risk for IHD in smokers compared with non-smokers. It is not completely clear whether or not this is a dose–response relationship, but it is apparent that cessation of smoking does lead to a fairly rapid decline in risk. Blood pressure is another independent risk factor for IHD. It has been demonstrated that there is a linear increase in risk as blood pressure, both systolic and diastolic, rises. Elevated blood pressure occurs in association with: smoking, alcohol consumption, dietary salt intake and body mass index. Blood cholesterol levels influence the risk of IHD, but with a more complex profile of risk. High levels of high-density lipoproteins (HDLs) are protective, but high levels of low-density lipoproteins (LDLs) and triglycerides are associated with increased risk.

Longitudinal studies have shown that the menopause causes several adverse effects on cardiovascular risk factors – lipid profiles in women become less favourable, there is a tendency to insulin resistance, an increased thrombotic tendency, and less favourable haemodynamic profiles – and these factors probably contribute to the increase in IHD. The menopause does not appear to have a direct effect on blood pressure.

HRT and IHD

Observational studies have suggested a reduction of 40–50% in the risk of IHD among healthy postmenopausal women taking oral unopposed oestrogens.[24] However, there has been one large meta-analysis of short-term oestrogen use, which found an increased risk of cardiovascular events in women taking hormone supplementation.[25] Furthermore, there are considerably less data from any clinical studies in which progestogens have been combined with oestrogens and it is now common practice for all non-hysterectomized women to have both hormones in order to reduce the risk of endometrial cancer. There is some evidence to suggest that progestogens may attenuate some of the favourable effects of oestrogens. There are, at present, no large randomized trials with IHD outcomes as the endpoints in healthy postmenopausal women, but there has been one large randomized, controlled trial of oestrogen/progestogen replacement therapy in women with established ischaemic heart disease (HERS trial).[26] This showed no reduction in the rate of myocardial infarction or heart-disease-related deaths in women taking HRT compared with women taking placebo, but there were increases in both the rates of gall bladder disease and thromboembolic events. It is possible that the results of the observational studies are subject to selection bias, i.e. those who choose oestrogens may have different health behaviours compared with women who do not choose them, with the implication that their risk for IHD may be different.[27] Therefore, whether or not HRT has an overall beneficial effect on an individual's risk of developing IHD is currently the subject of some controversy. There are two large randomized, controlled trials ongoing in Britain and the USA which will clarify this issue, but only after long-term follow-up, which will take several more years.

Chronic disease associated with HRT

Breast cancer

Until recently, breast cancer was the most common type of cancer affecting women (lung cancer has recently overtaken it), with 1 in 12 women affected. The frequency of breast cancer increases with age, so that it is common in postmenopausal women, and because it is a hormonal cancer the effects of hormone supplementation are of great concern to women.

A re-analysis of 51 studies was reported in 1997 which included 160 000 women, 52 000 with breast cancer.[28] The relative risk of developing breast cancer was increased by a factor of 1.023 for each year of use of HRT (*Table 2.3*). However, the effect was reduced after cessation of use of HRT, and almost completely disappeared after 5 years. Cancers diagnosed in women who had used HRT tended to be less clinically advanced at diagnosis. There was no additional effect from the type of HRT, or the dose prescribed, that could be detected. No differences in mortality from breast cancer in users of HRT compared with non-users were detected, but small studies have shown that the breast cancers in HRT users are better differentiated, with the possible implication that prognosis may be better.[29]

HRT and endometrial cancer

More than 30 observational studies have found that unopposed oestrogen therapy leads to an increase in endometrial cancer. This risk is directly related to dose, duration and type of oestrogen used and persists several years after discontinuing oestrogens.[30] Unopposed oestrogen for less than 5 years carries a threefold increase in risk, but long-term unopposed oestrogen may lead to a tenfold increase in risk. The addition of progesterones to oestrogens leads to endometrial atrophy, thereby almost entirely preventing the risk of endometrial cancer. All non-hysterectomized women are advised to have combination therapy.

HRT: the debate

Table 2.4 summarizes the lifetime risks for developing IHD, osteoporosis and hormonal cancers in women aged 50–94 years.

The menopause is associated with short-term troublesome symptoms, which can be effectively controlled by HRT. However, the menopause also represents a watershed, beyond which oestrogen deficiency leads to a steadily increasing risk of mortality and morbidity from IHD and osteoporosis. HRT does prevent bone loss and may prevent fractures in the elderly, but only if taken indefinitely. Furthermore, HRT does modify some risk factors for IHD, but the evidence

Table 2.3
Cumulative data for the risks of developing breast cancer with increased duration of use of HRT in women aged 50–70 years.

	Cumulative risk/1000 women
Never used HRT	45
HRT used for:	
5 years	47 (46–50)
10 years	51 (48–60)
15 years	57 (52–77)

Data from ref. 28.
HRT, hormone replacement therapy.

Table 2.4
Lifetime risks of mortality and morbidity for women aged 50–94 years.

IHD	Risk of death related to IHD	31%
Osteoporosis	Risk of death from hip fracture	2.8%
	Risk of hip fracture occurring	16%
	Risk of vertebral fracture occurring	32%
	Risk of wrist fracture occurring	15%
Cancers	Risk of death from breast cancer	2.8%
	Risk of death from endometrial cancer	0.7%

Data from ref. 31.
IHD, ischaemic heart disease.

that it reduces mortality from IHD is more controversial. However, both these diseases become most prevalent in the eighth decade of life and the benefits of HRT are only maintained whilst it is being taken; 20 or more years of HRT carry a significantly increased risk of breast cancer.

The debate is very complex; women vary in their uptake of, and compliance with, HRT. Observational studies suggest that those women who choose to take it do very well, with lower rates of mortality from all causes.[32] However, there is possibly a 'healthy user' effect. It may well be that HRT is the appropriate form of treatment for women with troublesome perimenopausal symptoms, to be taken only in the relatively short term. For the prevention of IHD and osteoporosis, until the results of the controlled trials are available, women must be given all the available information, and allowed to take a choice, based on their personal risk factors, fears and family histories. Breast cancer is less common than IHD overall, but in women aged less than 65 years breast cancer is more common than IHD. Women who are making decisions about HRT are typically in the age group that may have friends with breast cancer, but not IHD. Consequently, women are more likely to be adversely influenced by the small increase in risk of breast cancer than in the more favourable risk:benefit ratio of HRT overall, which may partly explain why compliance with HRT is very poor.[33]

Summary

The menopause has acquired considerable importance over the last century due to demographic changes. It is associated with perimenopausal symptoms, which can be troublesome, but HRT offers excellent palliation of these symptoms. The public health significance of the menopause lies in the association of oestrogen deficiency with osteoporosis and IHD, both major causes of mortality and morbidity in the elderly female population. HRT may have some potential in the prevention and treatment of these disorders, but it also has specific negative effects, such as breast and endometrial cancer, which are possibly significant enough to offset the benefits.

References

1. Davey DA. The menopause and climacteric. In: Whitfield CR (ed). *Dewhurst's Textbook of Obstetrics and Gynaecology for Postgraduates*, 5th edition. Blackwell Science: Oxford, 1995: 609–41.
2. Department of Health. *The Health of the Nation: One Year On.* HMSO: London, 1993.
3. Whitehead M, Godfree V. *The Menopause – a Growing Problem I. Hormone Replacement Therapy.* Churchill Livingstone: London, 1–6.
4. O'Neill TW, Silman AJ, Naves Diaz M, Cooper C, Kanis J, Felsenberg D and the European Vertebral Osteoporosis Study Group. Influence of hormonal and reproductive factors on the risk of vertebral deformity in European women. *Osteoporos Int* 1997; 7: 72–8.
5. Khaw KT. Epidemiology of the menopause. *Br Med Bull* 1992; **48**: 249–61.
6. McInlay SM, Brambilla DJ, Posner JG. The normal menopause transition. *Mauritas* 1992; **14**: 103–15.
7. Siddle N, Sarrel P, Whitehead M. The effect of hysterectomy on the age of ovarian failure: identification of a subgroup of women with premature loss of ovarian function and literature review. *Fertil Steril* 1987; **47**: 94–100.
8. Weg RB. Demography. In: Mishell DR Jr (ed). *Menopause: Physiology and Pharmacology.* Year Book Medical Publishers: Chicago, Ill, 1987: 23–40.

9. Greendale GA, Lee NP, Arriola ER. The menopause. *Lancet* 1999; **353**: 571–80.

10. Nicol-Smith L. Causality, menopause and depression: a critical review of the literature. *BMJ* 1996; **313**: 1229–32.

11. Consensus development conference: diagnosis, prophylaxis and treatment of osteoporosis. *Am J Med* 1993; **94**: 646–50.

12. Cooper C. Epidemiology and definition of osteoporosis. In: Compston J (ed). *Osteoporosis.* Royal College of Physicians of London: London, 1996: 1–10.

13. Melton LJ, Chrischilles EA, Cooper C, Lane AW, Riggs BL. How many women have osteoporosis? *J Bone Miner Res* 1992; 7: 1005–10.

14. Melton LJ. Perspectives: how many women have osteoporosis now? *J Bone Miner Res* 1995a; **41**: 57–64.

15. Petley GW, Cotton AM, Murrills AJ. Reference ranges of bone mineral density for women in southern England: the impact of local data on the diagnosis of osteoporosis. *Br J Radiol* 1996; **69**: 655–60.

16. Cooper C. The crippling consequences of fractures and their impact on quality of life. *Am J Med* 1997; **103**: 12S–19S.

17. Cooper C. Epidemiology and public health impact of osteoporosis. *Baillieres Clin Rheumatol* 1993; 7: 459–77.

18. O'Neill TW, Felsenberg D, Varlow J et al. The prevalence of vertebral deformity in European men and women: the European Vertebral Osteoporosis Study. *J Bone Miner Res* 1996; **11**: 1010–18.

19. Kaukonen JP, Karaharju EO, Porras M, Luthje P, Jakobsson A. Functional recovery after fracture of the distal forearm. *Ann Chir Gynaecol* 1988; 77: 27–31.

20. Grady D, Rubin SM, Petitti DB et al. Hormone therapy to prevent disease and prolong life in postmenopausal women. *Ann Intern Med* 1992; **117**: 1016–37.

21. Ettinger B, Grady D. The waning effect of postmenopausal estrogen therapy on osteoporosis. *N Engl J Med* 1993; **329**: 1192–3.

22. Schneider DL, Barrett-Connor EL, Morton DJ. Timing of postmenopausal estrogen for optimal bone mineral density. The Rancho Bernado study. *JAMA* 1997; **277**: 543–7.

23. Tunstall-Pedoe H. Cardiovascular diseases. In: Detels R, Holland W, McEwen J, Omenn G (eds). *Oxford Textbook of Public Health Medicine.* Oxford University Press: Oxford, 1997; **3**: 1021–42.

24. Barrett-Connor E, Grady D. Hormone replacement therapy, heart disease and other considerations. *Ann Rev Public Health* 1998; **19**: 55–72.

25. Hemminki E, McPherson K. Impact of postmenopausal hormone therapy on cardiovascular events and cancer: pooled data from clinical trials. *BMJ* 1997; **315**: 149–53.

26. Hulley S, Grady D, Bush T et al. for the Heart and Estrogen/Progestin Replacement Study (HERS) Research Group. Randomised trial of oestrogen plus progestin for secondary prevention of coronary heart disease in postmenopausal women. *JAMA* 1998; **280**: 605–13.

27. Posthuma WFM, Westendorp RGJ, Vandenbroucke JP. Cardioprotective effect of hormone replacement therapy in postmenopausal women: is the evidence biased? *BMJ* 1994; **308**: 1268–9.

28. Collaborative group on hormonal factors in breast cancer. Breast cancer and hormone replacement therapy: collaborative reanalysis

of data from 51 epidemiological studies of 52 705 women with breast cancer and 108 411 women without breast cancer. *Lancet* 1997; **350**: 1047–59.

29. Harding C, Knox WF, Faragher EB, Baildam A, Bindred NJ. Hormone replacement therapy and tumour grade in breast cancer: prospective study in screening unit. *BMJ* 1996; **312**: 1646–7.

30. Grady D, Gebretsadik T, Emster V, Petitti D. Hormone replacement therapy and endometrial cancer risk: a meta-analysis. *Obstet Gynecol* 1995; **85**: 304–12.

31. Cummings SR, Dennis DM, Rubin SM. Lifetime risk of hip, Colles', or vertebral fracture and coronary artery disease among white postmenopausal women. *Arch Intern Med* 1989; **149**: 2445–8.

32. Cauley JA, Seeley DG, Browner WS et al. Estrogen replacement therapy and mortality among older women. *Arch Intern Med* 1997; **157**: 2181–7.

33. Barrett-Connor E. Hormone replacement therapy. *BMJ* 1998; **317**: 457–61.

3

Mechanism of action of oestrogen and related compounds

George GJM Kuiper, Gert-Jan CM van den Bend, Johannes PTM van Leeuwen

The recent discovery that an additional oestrogen receptor (ERβ) subtype is present in many rat, mouse and human tissues has advanced our understanding of the mechanisms underlying oestrogen signalling. The existence of two oestrogen receptor subtypes (ERα and ERβ), their differential expression pattern and different actions on certain target gene promoters could provide explanations for the striking cell- and promoter-specific actions of oestrogen and selective oestrogen receptor modulators (SERMs).

Introduction

The steroid hormone oestrogen influences the growth, differentiation and function of peripheral tissues of the reproductive system such as mammary gland, uterus, vagina, ovary, testis, epididymis and prostate.[1] Oestrogen deficiency associated with menopause is the cause of the most rapid phase of bone loss in women, and oestrogen replacement therapy can prevent the fractures associated with bone loss.[2] A large and growing body of epidemiological data support biological effects of oestrogen on the cardiovascular system, resulting in protection from cardiovascular morbidity and mortality in women. These observations and experimental data obtained from certain animal models have led to the hypothesis that oestrogens exert direct effects upon the artery wall.[3] In the brain, oestrogen action affects both the activity and connectivity of certain neuronal populations, and thereby modulates physiological parameters important for animal reproduction, including mood and behaviour. Recent evidence suggests that oestrogen may also mediate non-reproductive events including learning and memory.[4] In addition, oestrogens are well known for their ability to promote the development of certain types of breast cancer. The oestrogen dependency of breast tumours is the key for the therapeutic intervention with oestrogen antagonists such as tamoxifen.[5,6]

Most of these very diverse effects of oestrogens are believed to be mediated by the so-called genomic pathway, involving the interaction of oestrogen with a nuclear receptor protein. An alternative non-genomic pathway, involving the interaction of oestrogen with putative cell membrane recognition sites, has been proposed as an explanation for the fast (<1 minute) and short-lived effects of oestrogen in the brain and in the reproductive system.[7] This chapter, however, will limit itself to the genomic pathway.

Oestrogens diffuse in and out of cells, but are retained in target cell nuclei by the oestrogen receptor protein (ER). Once bound by oestrogens, the ER undergoes a conformational change allowing the receptor to interact with high affinity with chromatin (***Figure 3.1***), and to modulate the expression of target genes.[1,6,8,9] The ER is a member of the nuclear hormone receptor family of genes, which also includes receptors for progestins, glucocorticoids, vitamin D and androgens.[1,10] These receptor proteins, which can all be regarded as ligand-regulated transcription factors, can be subdivided into several functional domains (***Figure 3.2***). The N-terminal A/B-domain is highly variable between different steroid receptors and contains a transactivation function called activation function-1 (AF-1). In fact, the ER contains at least two distinct activation functions: one is the already mentioned AF-1 and the second, AF-2, is located in the oestrogen-binding domain (E/F-domain). Via these activation functions the ER interacts with the components of the core transcriptional complex. Although the two activation functions have the potential to act independently, they appear to interact with each other in a way that is not yet completely understood.

The C-domain contains two zinc-binding clusters of amino acid residues, which are involved in specific DNA-binding by the ER. When activated by hormone binding the

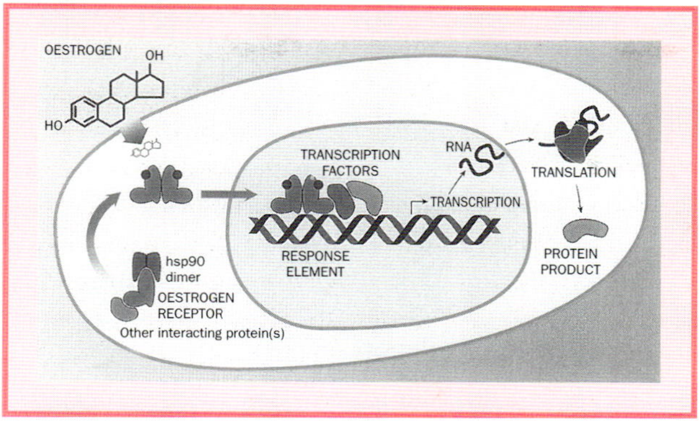

Figure 3.1
A model of oestrogen action. Oestrogens enter cells by simple or facilitated diffusion and bind to specific receptor proteins. The ER is a transcription factor that exists in an inactive state, either in the cytoplasm or nucleus, complexed with heat shock protein 90 and possibly other proteins as well. Upon oestrogen binding, the receptor undergoes an ill-defined activation step called transformation, which enables it to bind to cognate DNA response elements in target gene promoters. Subsequently, recruitment of co-activators and general transcription factors results in the formation of an active transcriptional complex and enhancement of target gene transcription.

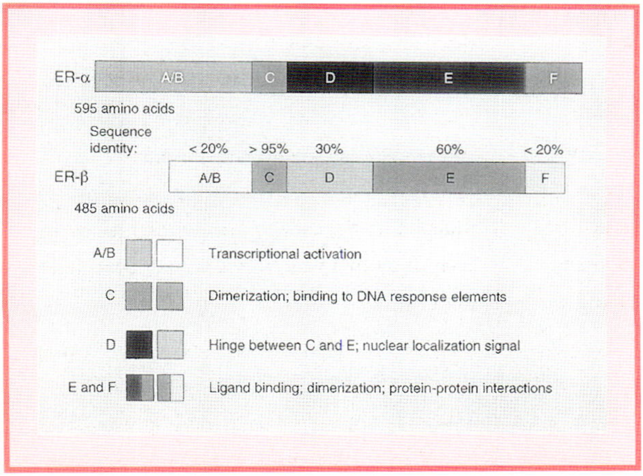

Figure 3.2
ER subtypes. ER subtypes α and β possess the same functional domains and appear to bind the same ligands, although in some cases with different affinities. The aminoterminal A/B-domain (AF-1 function) has the least amino acid sequence identity, while the C-domain (DNA-binding) has the highest amino acid sequence identity.

ER binds to specific DNA sequences, termed oestrogen response elements (EREs), found in the vicinity of target genes. Oestrogen response elements consist of inverted repeats of the sequence A/GGGTCA separated by three nucleotides, and the ER binds to these elements as a dimer. In addition, it is now evident that ERs are capable of regulating the transcription of genes that lack EREs in their promoter region by modulating the activity of other transcription factors such as AP-1, NF-κB and Sp1.[11–13] In fact, it is likely that the transcription of many ER target genes is regulated by these indirect or 'non-classical' mechanisms.

The E/F domain or ligand-binding domain is functionally complex because it contains regions important for ligand binding and ER dimerization as well as the AF-2 function. The crystal structure of the ligand-binding domain of the ER has been solved,[8,9] both as a complex with oestrogen or with SERMs (selective oestrogen receptor modulators) such as tamoxifen and raloxifene. It appears that a major role of ligand binding is an alteration in the conformation of the ligand-binding domain, creating novel surfaces by which the ER interacts with co-activators and possibly other regulatory proteins. These novel interaction surfaces are an important part of the AF-2 function. Gene transcription depends on the formation of a pre-initiation complex that includes basal transcription factors, and one of the roles of the ER is thought to be the stabilization of this complex. In recent years it has become evident that the ER interacts via its AF-2 in a ligand-dependent manner with the basal transcription complex via 'bridging proteins' called co-activators. A detailed description of all co-activators, their characteristics and mechanism of action, is beyond the scope of this chapter; however, they are described in depth elsewhere.[14–16]

The ER-encoding cDNAs were cloned during the period 1986–87 from several species.[1,6] Since that time it has been generally accepted that only one ER gene exists, although this assumption made it difficult to understand completely the complicated pharmacology and tissue selectivity of synthetic oestrogens and SERMs in vivo, as well as the differential effects of these compounds in a variety of cell lines.[17,18] At the end of 1995, a second ER-encoding cDNA was cloned (ERβ) and therefore the previously cloned ER was renamed ERα.[19–23] When compared with ERα, the protein sequence of ERβ demonstrates considerable homology in the DNA- and ligand-binding domains (***Figure 3.2***). Evaluation of the binding affinities of a variety of synthetic and naturally occurring oestrogenic compounds (including phytoestrogens and environmental oestrogenic compounds) has shown that the relative binding affinities for ERα and ERβ are very similar.[24,25] Also, the SERMs tamoxifen, raloxifene and ICI-164,384 have

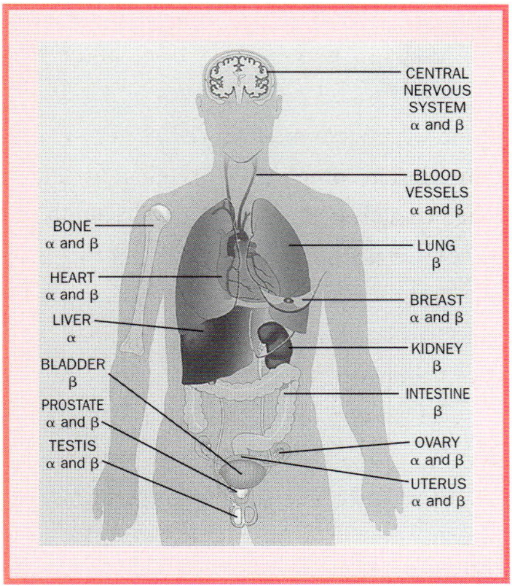

Figure 3.3
Distribution of human ER subtypes. This distribution is mainly based on the measurement of ER mRNA levels. The pattern awaits confirmation at the protein level when subtype-specific monoclonal antibodies become available.

similar affinities for both ER subtypes.[25]

The transcriptional activity of ERs is usually measured in so-called transactivation assays. In these assays the ER is transiently expressed in heterologous cells together with a plasmid containing an ERE linked to a reporter gene, such as chloramphenicol acetyltransferase or luciferase. After incubation of the cells with ligand (oestrogen or SERMs) the enzyme activity of the reporter gene is determined, and is a measure of the ER transcriptional activity. In these transactivation assays it was shown that ERβ is able to mediate the effects of oestrogen in a dose-dependent manner, and that this activity can be significantly reduced by the addition of known ERα antagonists such as tamoxifen, raloxifene and ICI-164,384/ICI-182,780.[19–21,26] In other words, the ERβ protein is a genuine oestrogen receptor protein.

Expression of ERα and ERβ

The presence of ERs has been demonstrated in numerous normal and pathological tissues, and many genes regulated by oestrogen in a tissue-specific manner have been identified.[27] Various methods have been used to study ER expression including ligand-binding assays and steroid autoradiography, immunocytochemistry, and molecular biological methods such as reverse transcriptase polymerase chain reaction, northern blotting and in situ hybridization.[1,6,24,27,28] Because ERβ was discovered quite recently, no specific monoclonal antibodies that can be used consistently for immunohistochemistry on a wide range of normal and pathological tissues are yet available. In the past, various polyclonal and monoclonal antibodies to the ER protein have been developed, but it has been established in retrospect that most of these only recognize the ERα protein (G. Kuiper, unpublished observations). Our current

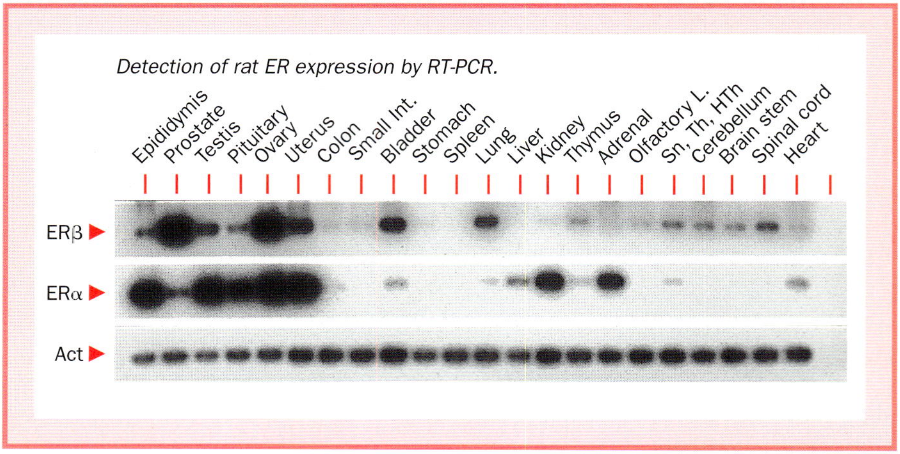

Figure 3.4
Rat transcript tissue distribution of ERα and ERβ. Male and female rats (6–8 weeks old) were killed by cervical dislocation and tissues were collected. Tissue samples were immediately processed for total RNA isolation, and random-hexamer-primed cDNA synthesis was performed. For the PCR amplification 5% of the synthesized cDNA was added to PCR reaction mixtures containing oligonucleotide primers specific for ERα, ERβ, or actin. After agarose gel electrophoresis and blotting to nitrocellulose filters the PCR products were hybridized to specific internal oligonucleotide probes. All tissues shown were from male rats except for the female tissues such as uterus and ovary. The RNA isolated from pancreas and brain cortex appeared degraded and was discarded. Abbreviations: Sn, substantia nigra and preopticus; Th, thalamus; Hth, hypothalamus; olfactory L., olfactory lobe; small int., small intestines. Based on ref. 24.

knowledge of the distribution of ERα and ERβ is therefore based on mRNA analysis either by reverse transcriptase polymerase chain reaction, northern blotting or by in situ hybridization, and the relative levels of ERα and ERβ protein have yet to be determined.[19–22,24,28,29]

Expression of human ERα and ERβ has been found in the central nervous system, blood vessels, mammary gland, uterus, bone, lung, kidney, intestine, ovary, prostate, bladder, epididymis and testis (***Figure 3.3***). In rodents, a broadly similar distribution was found (***Figure 3.4***). In more detailed studies it appeared that in various instances in which organs express both ER subtypes the ERs are expressed in different cell-types. This might indicate that ERα and ERβ have distinct functions in some instances.

An interesting example is the rodent brain. Through the use of in situ hybridization, the distributions of ERα- and ERβ-mRNA have been evaluated in adjacent sections of the rat brain.[28] When compared with ERα-mRNA, ERβ-mRNA containing perikarya were more widely distributed throughout the brain, while considerable overlap was seen in the preoptic area, the bed nucleus of stria terminalis and throughout the lower brain stem.[28] Based on the distribution of ERβ in the rodent brain, it is likely that the hormonal actions mediated by ERβ regulate many important neuronal functions. Some of these functions were known to be regulated by oestrogen, although little or no ER (read ERα) was found in these regions. For example, the role of oestrogen in cognitive functions is supported by recent observations that oestrogen replacement therapy improves cognitive functions in postmenopausal women.[4,30] Until the discovery of ERβ and its localization in regions associated with learning and memory (neocortex, hippocampus and nuclei of the basal forebrain[28]), these data were difficult to explain because ERα is sparse or absent in these regions. On the other hand, the lack of neurons expressing ERβ-mRNA in the ventromedial hypothalamic nucleus[28] and the low level of expression in the arcuate nucleus suggest that ERβ, unlike ERα, may play only a limited role in the central regulation of procreation. Thus, the differential distribution of ER subtypes in the brain may provide a mechanism for the selective modulation (by existing or novel ER subtype selective ligands) of physiological parameters involved with reproductive as well as regulation of non-reproductive events.

Bone is another example of an oestrogen-regulated tissue in which ERα and ERβ might have different roles. In primary osteoblastic cells isolated from the bone of neonatal rats, both ERα- and ERβ-mRNA were detected, although the level of ERβ-mRNA was much higher than that of ERα-mRNA.[31] This difference in expression level was also found by in situ hybridization studies with ERα- and ERβ-specific riboprobes on rat bone, in which ERβ was detected in osteoblasts whereas ERα was not detected (S. Windahl, G. Kuiper, G. Andersson, unpublished observations). Also, the differential regulation of ERα- and ERβ-mRNA during the proliferation, differentiation and mineralization phase of the human foetal osteoblastic cell line SV-HFO suggests an additional function for the role of ERβ to ERα in bone metabolism.[32]

In the cardiovascular system also the ER subtypes might have different roles. Although women generally possess a significantly greater incidence of multiple risk factors associated with cardiovascular diseases, such as obesity, elevated blood pressure, high plasma cholesterol levels and diabetes, their risk of developing this disease is significantly lower than that of men of a similar age.[3] At menopause the decline in oestrogens is accompanied by an increased incidence of cardiovascular diseases, and long-term oestrogen replacement therapy delays cardiovascular disease development.[33] The putative so-called vasculoprotective effect of oestrogen has indeed been documented in more detail in experimental animal models. Oestrogen has been found to inhibit the intimal thickening after mechanical carotid injury in rabbits, rats and mice.[3] Both ERα and ERβ are expressed in the endothelium and smooth muscle cells of arteries in various species.[29,34,35] Interestingly, in the mouse carotid injury model, the oestrogen-induced inhibition of vascular smooth muscle cell proliferation after vessel wall damage was similar in wild-type and ERα-deficient mice,[36] thus indicating the existence of an ERα-independent mechanism. In support of this hypothesis, in situ hybridization studies showed that ERβ-mRNA but not ERα-mRNA is markedly induced in the aortae of rats following balloon injury.[35] Compounds that selectively activate ERβ may be good candidates in the search for vasculoselective oestrogens, provided that undesirable side-effects, such as endometrial stimulation, can be avoided.[37]

Tissue-specific effects of oestrogen and SERMs

Most drugs targeted at the ER, such as tamoxifen, ICI-164,384/ICI-182,780 and raloxifene (known as SERM), exhibit a curious pharmacological profile, acting as either oestrogen antagonist or agonist depending on the species, tissue and the dose administered.[6,8,9,17,18] An agonist mimics the action of the cognate ligand oestrogen, whereas an antagonist counteracts the oestrogen action. A mixed agonist–antagonist partially inhibits the action of an agonist but also partially mimics the response of the agonist. The benzothiophene analogue raloxifene has been reported to act as an oestrogen antagonist in breast tumour tissue and the brain, while it has potentially beneficial oestrogen-like effects in bone and in modulating factors associated with cardiovascular diseases.[38,39] Another example is tamoxifen, which was developed as an oestrogen antagonist for the treatment of breast cancer and subsequently shown to have oestrogen-like effects on bone and in the cardiovascular system.[5,6,17] However, the potentially beneficial effects of tamoxifen in reducing the risk of osteoporotic fractures and coronary heart disease in postmenopausal women are at least partially offset by oestrogenic effects on the uterus, increased risk of endometrial cancer development, and antagonistic activity in the brain.[5]

Tamoxifen and raloxifene are examples of mixed agonist–antagonists of oestrogen action. The definition of whether a compound is an agonist or antagonist is only appropriate in the context of a certain response. The existence of mixed agonists–antagonists of oestrogen action shows that the model of ER action in which ligand is responsible for

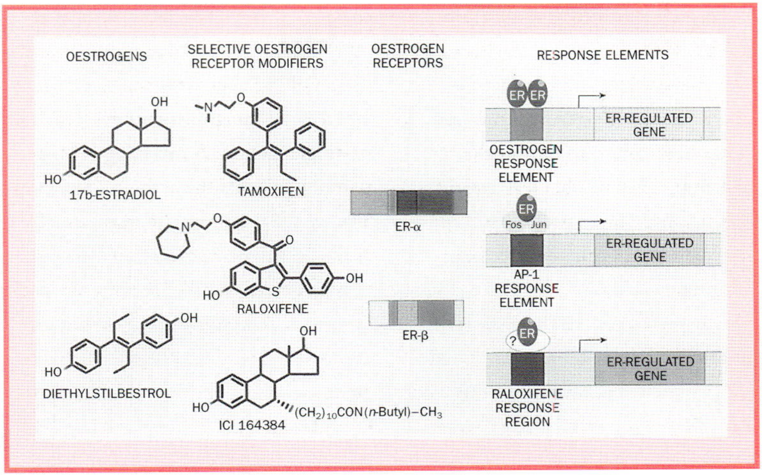

Figure 3.5
Selective modulation of oestrogen receptor action. The naturally occurring oestrogen is a C18 steroid, characterized by the presence of an aromatic A ring, a phenolic hydroxyl group at C-3, and a hydroxyl group at position 17β of the D ring. Many synthetic compounds with phenolic ring structures mimic oestrogen action: an example is diethylstilbestrol. The stilbene ring structure of diethylstilbestrol is the chemical basis of several triphenylethylene compounds that possess antioestrogenic activity: examples are tamoxifen and raloxifene. Remarkably, antioestrogenic activity is also shown by 7α-substituents of oestrogen, such as ICI-164,384. The liganded oestrogen receptor, either ERα or ERβ, is able to bind to DNA response elements either directly or 'indirectly' via protein–protein interactions with other DNA-bound transcription factors, such as AP-1.

switching the ER from an inactive state to an active state is an oversimplification. It is clear now that different ligands/SERMs induce different conformational changes in the ligand-binding domain.[8,9] Various 'activity states' of the ER exist and the biological activity of a certain ligand/SERM is influenced by many factors, such as the cell and promoter context of the DNA-bound receptor.[8,9,18] Different ligands/SERMs acting through the same ER may display different activities in different tissues, and therefore the name SERM (selective oestrogen receptor modulator) is used to describe these compounds. Exactly how SERMs exert their tissue-selective effects is the subject of much speculation and research (*Figure 3.5*). Throughout the years various models have been provided.

Activation function-1 versus activation function-2

As already mentioned, the ER has at least two

regions which are required for maximal transcriptional activity in the presence of oestrogen: activating function-1 (AF-1) located in the N-terminal A/B-domain and activation function-2 (AF-2) located within the ligand-binding domain. In various studies it has been shown that AF-1 and AF-2 function in a cell-specific manner, depending on the target gene promoter context.[17,18,26,40] It was hypothesized that, depending on the promoter context, either or both AFs may be required, and different compounds could differentially affect the interaction of these AFs with the transcriptional apparatus. Especially in the case of the mixed agonist–antagonist tamoxifen this hypothesis was confirmed. It was found that in cell lines where AF-2 and AF-1 are required for ER transcriptional activity (as for instance in breast tumour cells) tamoxifen acts as an antagonist on ERE-reporter gene constructs, whereas in cell lines in which AF-1 alone is sufficient (for instance in endometrial tumour cells) tamoxifen acts as an agonist.[17] Thus, tamoxifen was defined as an AF-1 agonist and an AF-2 antagonist in these experiments. For ERα, but not for ERβ, agonistic activity on ERE-reporter gene constructs in various cell lines in the presence of tamoxifen has been described.[26,40,41] The A/B-regions of ERα and ERβ are poorly conserved (only 20% amino acid homology), suggesting that their AF-1 activities might be different, and possibly that they contact the transcriptional apparatus in a different manner. Upon replacing the A/B region of ERβ with the A/B region of ERα, this mutant ERα/β chimera protein is now able to activate transcription in the presence of tamoxifen, while wild-type ERβ protein is not.[41] In other words, the agonistic activity of tamoxifen in certain cell and promoter contexts is mediated by the AF-1 function of ERα, and is not supported by the AF-1 function of ERβ. At the moment it is unknown which unique feature of the AF-1 function of ERα is responsible for the described agonistic activity of tamoxifen. Together, the differences in the AF-1 function of ERα and ERβ and the differential expression pattern of ERα and ERβ could contribute to the mixed agonist–antagonist profile of tamoxifen. This is an important conclusion because it indicates that cell- or tissue-restricted agonists/antagonists can be developed.

Various AF-1 agonists, such as tamoxifen, nafoxidine and clomiphene, have oestrogen-like activity in bone.[42] It was predicted therefore that compounds that have cell-type specific AF-1 agonistic activity (on ERα) function as an oestrogen agonist in bone. It soon appeared that this assumption is not true because it was found that raloxifene does prevent the ovariectomy-induced bone loss in rats, but has only minimal or no AF-1-mediated agonistic activity on ERE-reported gene constructs in any cell line tested.[26,42] Raloxifene has a similar pharmaceutical profile to tamoxifen in all tissues except the uterus, where it demonstrates no oestrogen-like activity.[38,39] The lack of a strict association between oestrogen-like activity in bone and uterus and AF-1-mediated activity on ERE-reported gene constructs indicated that alternative pathways of ER action could exist.

Alternative response elements

Raloxifene, like tamoxifen, counters oestrogenic effects in breast while acting like oestrogen in bone. But, raloxifene does not promote excess growth of uterine tissue, implying that it could be used to combat osteoporosis without increasing the risk of developing breast cancer or endometrial cancer.

An important key to the mechanism of action of raloxifene in bone was the finding that raloxifene activates the gene encoding transforming growth factor-β3 (TGFβ3), a protein considered important to keep bones strong in animals.[43] Also, oestrogen activates the TGFβ3 gene, but in a much less efficient way compared with raloxifene. The promoter region of the TGFβ3 gene does not contain a 'classical' ERE, but a different sequence (called the raloxifene response region) to which the ERα protein binds indirectly[43] (see also ***Figure 3.5***). One or more additional proteins, interacting with ERα, are needed to link the ERα–raloxifene complex to the DNA. These proteins have not been identified so far. It appears that the effects of SERMs like raloxifene can be mediated in certain cells and on certain promoters by pathways other than via the ER–ERE complex, thus providing yet another possible explanation for the tissue-selective effects of SERMs.

An even more surprising finding was the discovery of genes that showed 'reversed pharmacology', i.e. induced in ER-containing cells by SERM treatment and suppressed when the ER is occupied with the physiological ligand oestrogen.[44,45] It was found that tamoxifen and its main metabolite 4-OH-tamoxifen increase the expression of quinone-reductase (a phase II detoxification enzyme) in breast cancer cells, while oestrogen suppresses this increase.[44] More detailed experiments, involving transient transfections of breast cancer cells with ERα or ERβ expression vectors and a reporter gene construct consisting of a part of the quinone reductase gene promoter, showed that both ERα and ERβ increased reporter gene activity in the presence of tamoxifen, but did not increase activity in the presence of oestrogen.[45] The quinone reductase gene promoter does not contain a 'classical' ERE, and the exact DNA sequence element(s) mediating SERM responsiveness have not been identified to date. It has been proposed that tamoxifen may function as an anticancer drug, partly by acting as an antioxidant.[5] The induction of quinone reductase activity by tamoxifen in breast epithelial cells might protect against the toxic effects of certain carcinogens.

Another example of non-ERE-mediated gene expression by ERs is the action of ERα and ERβ at AP-1 enhancer elements.[46] Both ER subtypes mediate gene transcription from AP-1 enhancer elements, which require ligand and the AP-1 transcription factors *Fos* and *Jun* for transcription activation.[11] Interestingly, in transient transfection systems, ERα and ERβ, when complexed with oestrogen, were shown to signal in opposite ways from an AP-1 site in the context of the collagenase promoter with oestrogen activating transcription in the presence of ERα and inhibiting transcription in the presence of ERβ. The SERMs tamoxifen, raloxifene and ICI-164,384 were activators with ERβ as well as with ERα, although the degree of stimulation differed between cell types.[46] Thus, the role of oestrogen complexed to ERβ appears to be to turn off transcription from AP-1 elements whereas SERMs may override this blockade and activate transcription.

The finding that SERMs can activate via ERα and/or ERβ the expression in some cells of certain genes, which do not contain ERE-elements in their promoter regions, provides an important explanation for the tissue-selective effects of SERMs. It can be anticipated that in the future more genes regulated by SERMs will be identified. All the mechanisms described so far as explanations for the tissue-selective effects of SERMs are by no means mutually exclusive or complete. The great challenge of the future will be to use our rapidly increasing knowledge on the mechanism of action of ERs and SERMs in a rational manner for the development of the next generation of ER-targeted drugs with yet further improved therapeutic profiles.

Final comments

Since the discovery of ERβ, we have found that the expression patterns of the ER subtypes differ within tissues.[22,24,28,29] The differential expression of ERα and ERβ could be regarded as support for the hypothesis that the ER subtype proteins have different functions, although some overlap may occur. In other words, ERβ is not a backup of ERα and vice versa.

More detailed information about the physiological importance of ERα and ERβ might come from the characteristics of mice lacking either functional ERα or ERβ. A mutant mouse line without a functional ERα protein (ERKO) has been created and assessed for oestrogenic responses.[47,48] Female ERKO mice are infertile and show hypoplastic uteri and hyperaemic ovaries with no detectable corpora lutea. The mammary glands of ERKO animals are underdeveloped, and it remains to be established if this is caused by the absence of ERα in the mammary gland itself or due to alterations in circulating levels of prolactin and/or growth hormone. Adult male ERKO mice have a reduced testis size and are infertile.[48,49] While the ERKO mice displayed many of the characteristics expected from an oestrogen-insensitive animal, there are examples of oestrogen-regulated systems that are not or are only partially affected.[36,50,51] Recently, a mutant mouse line without a functional ERβ protein (BERKO) was created.[52] Breeding experiments with young sexually mature BERKO females show that they are fertile and exhibit normal sexual behaviour, but have fewer and smaller litters than wild-type mice. Superovulation experiments indicated that this reduction in fertility is the result of reduced ovarian efficiency. The BERKO females have normal breast development and lactate normally. Young, sexually mature male BERKO mice showed no overt abnormalities and reproduced normally. Older males, on the other hand, displayed signs of prostatic hyperplasia. Although the comparative characterization of ERKO and BERKO mice is far from complete, the fact that the phenotypes are already so different points again in the direction that ERα and ERβ have different physiological roles. Obviously, the lack of ERα cannot be compensated by ERβ or vice versa. Much future work is needed to determine the effects of the absence of ERα or ERβ in ageing animals, particularly in relation to the cardiovascular system, brain function and bone homeostasis.

So far, only one germline mutation of the human ERα gene associated with disease has been identified.[53] This male patient suffered from osteoporosis, unfused epiphyses, and continued linear growth in adulthood. Do germline mutations of the human ERβ gene exist and which diseases are associated with them? Are they associated with infertility, osteoporosis, cardiovascular or neurodegenerative diseases? Perhaps further characterization of the BERKO mouse model could help to elucidate the importance of ERβ in disease, and guide us in selecting patients with a suspected ERβ mutation.

The ERα and ERβ proteins can form heterodimers on consensus EREs in vitro,[23,54–57] but it is unknown to what extent heterodimers really exist in vivo and what their activity could be (***Figure 3.6***). Do target genes exist that are exclusively regulated by the heterodimer instead of by the respective homodimers? In addition, do ERα and ERβ homodimers interact differentially with different EREs within the context of target gene promoters? Both ERα and ERβ bind to the consensus ERE (GGTCANNNTGACC), but this sequence only mediates the expression of a single endogenous gene (i.e. vitellogenin). All other EREs identified to date have one or more base changes from the consensus sequence; the most common motif being one half-site identical to that in the vitellogenin-ERE and a second half-site with considerable variability in nucleotide sequence.[58,59] Differential binding and activation by ERα

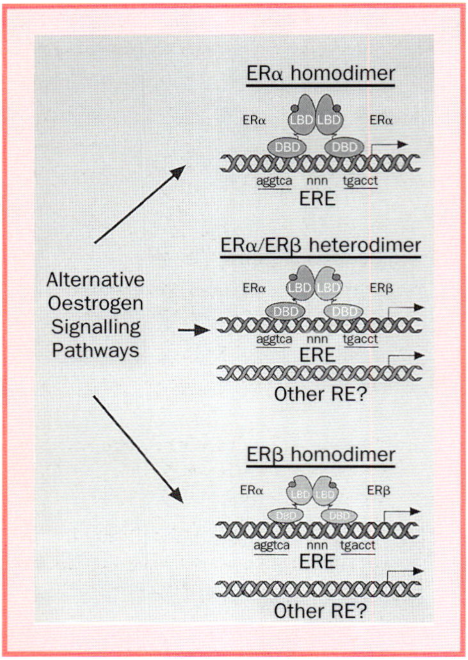

Figure 3.6
Alternative oestrogen signalling pathways. The existence of two ER subtypes and their ability to form DNA-binding heterodimers suggests the existence of three potential pathways of oestrogen signalling. In cells expressing only the ERα or ERβ subtype homodimers of either subtype can interact with response elements in target gene promoters and influence transcription levels. In cells expressing both subtypes, heterodimers can be formed depending on the ratio of subtypes. It cannot be excluded at this stage that unique response elements exist within the context of target gene promoters which interact preferentially with ERβ homodimers or ERα/ERβ heterodimers. An open question in this regard is whether oestrogen target genes exist which are exclusively regulated by either of the homodimers or the heterodimer.

and ERβ when linked to different EREs has indeed been described in vitro.[58,59] This raises the possibility that different target cells may respond differently to the same hormonal stimulus due to alternative expression of ER subtypes. Varying ratios of the ERα and ERβ protein within different cells, resulting in different populations of homo- and heterodimers, could constitute a hitherto unrecognized mechanism involved in the tissue- and cell-specific action of oestrogens and SERMs.[56]

Oestrogen replacement therapy in postmenopausal women is used increasingly with the aim of relieving hot flushes and mood changes, reducing skin and reproductive tract atrophy, and delaying atherosclerosis, the loss of bone mass and neurodegeneration.[33,60] The most compelling problem is the increased risk of breast and endometrial cancer and inconvenience due to irregular spotting and bleeding. Given the low expression level of ERβ compared with ERα in the uterus, an ERβ-selective SERM may be less prone to causing spotting and bleeding. At the same time, given the relatively high expression of ERβ in the cerebral cortex and hippocampus of the brain as well as in bone, such compounds could be beneficial for preventing loss of cognitive function and bone mass. While this may be wishful thinking at the moment, attempts to develop ERβ-selective ligands are well underway[26,60,61] and it may not be too long before this prediction can be tested.

Finally, do we have all the ERs? Is there an ERγ yet to be discovered? Whether an ERγ exists or not, the discovery of ERβ has demonstrated that the mechanism of oestrogen and SERM action is much more complicated than was ever anticipated. Almost 40 years after the initial description of the mechanism of oestrogen action[62,63] it appears that we are at the start of renewed explorations.

References

1. Tsai M-J, Clark JH, Schrader WT, O'Malley BW. Mechanisms of action of hormones that act as transcription factors. In: Wilson JD, Foster DW, Kronenberg HM, Larsen PR (eds). *Textbook of Endocrinology*, 9th edition. WB Saunders: Philadelphia, 1998: 55–94.
2. Riggs BL, Khosla S, Melton J. A unitary model for involutional osteoporosis: estrogen deficiency causes both type I and type II osteoporosis in postmenopausal women and contributes to bone loss in aging men. *J Bone Miner Res* 1998; **13**: 763–73.
3. Farhat MY, Lavigne MC, Ramwell PW. The vascular protective effects of estrogen. *FASEB J* 1996; **10**: 615–24.
4. Tang M-X, Jacobs D, Stern Y et al. Effect of oestrogen during menopause on risk and age at onset of Alzheimer's disease. *Lancet* 1996; **348**: 429–32.
5. Jordan VC. Tamoxifen: toxicities and drug resistance during the treatment and prevention of breast cancer. *Annu Rev Pharmacol Toxicol* 1995; **35**: 195–211.
6. Jensen EV. Steroid hormones, receptors and antagonists. *Ann N Y Acad Sci* 1996; **784**: 1–17.
7. Wehling M. Specific, nongenomic actions of steroid hormones. *Annu Rev Physiol* 1997; **59**: 365–93.
8. Brzozowski AM, Pike ACW, Dauter Z et al. Molecular basis of agonism and antagonism in the oestrogen receptor. *Nature* 1997; **389**: 753–8.
9. Shiau AK, Barstad D, Loria PM et al. The structural basis of estrogen receptor/coactivator recognition and the antagonism of this interaction by tamoxifen. *Cell* 1998; **95**: 927–37.
10. White R, Parker MG. Molecular mechanisms of steroid hormone action. *Endocrine-Related Cancer* 1998; **5**: 1–14.
11. Gaub M-P, Bellard M, Scheuer I et al. Activation of the ovalbumin gene by the estrogen receptor involves the fos–jun complex. *Cell* 1990; **63**: 1267–76.
12. Stein B, Yang MX. Repression of the interleukin-6 promoter by estrogen receptor is mediated by NF-κB and C/EBP. *Mol Cell Biol* 1995; **15**: 4971–9.
13. Porter W, Saville B, Hoivik D, Safe S. Functional synergy between the transcription

factor Sp1 and the estrogen receptor. *Mol Endocrinol* 1997; **11**: 1569–80.

14. Jenster G. Coactivators and corepressors as mediators of nuclear receptor function: an update. *Mol Cell Endocrinol* 1998; **143**: 1–7.

15. Klein-Hitpass L, Schwerk C, Kahmann S, Vaßen L. Targets of activated steroid hormone receptors: basal transcription factors and receptor interacting proteins. *J Mol Med* 1998; **76**: 490–6.

16. Horwitz KB, Jackson TA, Bain DL et al. Nuclear receptor coactivators and corepressors. *Mol Endocrinol* 1996; **10**: 1167–76.

17. Katzenellenbogen JA, O'Malley BW, Katzenellenbogen BS. Tripartite steroid hormone receptor pharmacology: interaction with multiple effector sites as a basis for the cell- and promoter-specific action of these hormones. *Mol Endocrinol* 1996; **10**: 119–31.

18. McDonnell DP, Clemm DL, Hermann T et al. Analysis of estrogen receptor function in vitro reveals three distinct classes of antiestrogens. *Mol Endocrinol* 1995; **9**: 659–69.

19. Kuiper GGJM, Enmark E, Pelto-Huikko M et al. Cloning of a novel estrogen receptor expressed in rat prostate and ovary. *Proc Natl Acad Sci U S A* 1996; **93**: 5925–30.

20. Mosselman S, Polman J, Dijkema R. ERβ: identification and characterization of a novel human estrogen receptor. *FEBS Lett* 1996; **392**: 49–53.

21. Tremblay GB, Tremblay A, Copeland NG et al. Cloning, chromosomal localization, and functional analysis of the murine estrogen receptor β. *Mol Endocrinol* 1997; **11**: 353–65.

22. Enmark E, Pelto-Huikko M, Grandien K et al. Human estrogen receptor β-gene structure, chromosomal localization and expression pattern. *J Clin Endocrinol Metab* 1997; **82**: 4258–65.

23. Ogawa S, Inoue S, Watanabe T et al. The complete primary structure of human estrogen receptor-β and its heterodimerization with estrogen receptor-α in vivo and in vitro. *Biochem Biophys Res Commun* 1998; **243**: 122–6.

24. Kuiper GGJM, Carlsson B, Grandien K et al. Comparison of the ligand binding specificity and transcript tissue distribution of estrogen receptors α and β. *Endocrinology* 1997; **138**: 863–70.

25. Kuiper GGJM, Lemmen JG, Carlsson B et al. Interaction of estrogenic chemicals and phytoestrogens with estrogen receptor β. *Endocrinology* 1998; **139**: 4252–63.

26. Barkhem T, Carlsson B, Nilsson Y et al. Differential response of estrogen receptor β and estrogen receptor α to partial estrogen agonists/antagonists. *Mol Pharmacol* 1998; **54**: 105–12.

27. Ciocca DR, Vargas-Roig LM. Estrogen receptors in human nontarget tissues: biological and clinical implications. *Endocr Rev* 1995; **16**: 35–62.

28. Kuiper GGJM, Shughrue PJ, Merchenthaler I, Gustafsson J-Å. The estrogen receptor β subtype: a novel mediator of estrogen action in neuroendocrine systems. *Front Neuroendocrinol* 1998; **19**: 253–86.

29. Pau CY, Pau K-Y, Spies HG. Putative estrogen receptor β and α mRNA expression in male and female rhesus macaques. *Mol Cell Endocrinol* 1998; **146**: 59–68.

30. Birge SJ. Is there a role for oestrogen replacement therapy in the prevention and treatment of dementia? *J Am Geriatr Soc* 1996; **44**: 865–70.

31. Onoe Y, Miyaura C, Ohta H et al. Expression of estrogen receptor β in rat bone. *Endocrinology* 1997; **138**: 4509–12.

32. Arts J, Kuiper GGJM, Janssen JMMF et al. Differential expression of estrogen receptors α and β mRNA during differentiation of human osteoblast SV-HFO cells. *Endocrinology* 1997; **138**: 5067–70.

33. Lamberts SWJ, van den Beld AW, van der Lely A-J. The endocrinology of aging. *Science* 1997; **278**: 419–24.

34. Register TC, Adams MR. Coronary artery and cultured aortic smooth muscle cells express mRNA for both the classical estrogen receptor and the newly described estrogen receptor β. *J Steroid Biochem Mol Biol* 1998; **64**: 187–91.

35. Kim SK, Lindner V, Karas RH et al. Expression of estrogen receptor β mRNA in normal and injured blood vessels. *Circ Res* 1998; **83**: 224–9.

36. Iafrati MD, Karas RH, Aronovitz M et al. Estrogen inhibits the vascular injury response in estrogen receptor α-deficient mice. *Nat Med* 1997; **3**: 545–8.

37. Mäkelä S, Savolainen H, Aavik E et al. Differentiation between vasculoprotective and uterotrophic effects of ligands with different binding affinities to estrogen receptors α and β. *Proc Natl Acad Sci USA* 1999; **96**: 7077–82.

38. Delmas PD, Bjarnasan NH, Mitlak BH et al. Effects of raloxifene on bone mineral density, serum cholesterol concentration, and uterine endometrium in postmenopausal women. *N Engl J Med* 1997; **337**: 1641–7.

39. Gustafsson J-Å. Raloxifene: magic bullet for heart and bone? *Nat Med* 1998; **4**: 152–3.

40. Watanabe T, Inoue S, Ogawa S et al. Agonistic effect of tamoxifen is dependent on cell type, ERE promoter context, and estrogen receptor subtype: functional difference between estrogen receptors α and β. *Biochem Biophys Res Commun* 1997; **236**: 140–5.

41. McInerney EM, Weis KE, Sun J et al. Transcription activation by the human estrogen receptor subtype β studied with ERβ and ERα receptor chimeras. *Endocrinology* 1998; **139**: 4513–22.

42. Sato M, Rippy MK, Bryant HU. Raloxifene, tamoxifen, nafoxidine, or estrogen effects on reproductive and nonreproductive tissues in ovariectomized rats. *FASEB J* 1996; **10**: 905–12.

43. Yang NN, Venugopalan M, Hardikar S, Glasebrook A. Identification of an estrogen response element activated by metabolites of estradiol and raloxifen. *Science* 1996; **273**: 1222–5 (erratum: **275**: 1249).

44. Montano MM, Katzenellenbogen BS. The quinone reductase gene: a unique estrogen receptor-regulated gene that is activated by antiestrogens. *Proc Natl Acad Sci U S A* 1997; **94**: 2581–6.

45. Montano MM, Jaiswal AK, Katzenellenbogen BS. Transcriptional regulation of the human quinone reductase gene by antiestrogen-liganded estrogen receptor-α and estrogen receptor-β. *J Biol Chem* 1998; **273**: 25 443–9.

46. Paech K, Webb P, Kuiper GGJM et al. Differential ligand activation of estrogen receptors ERα and ERβ at AP1 sites. *Science* 1997; **277**: 1508–10.

47. Lubahn DB, Moyer JS, Golding TS et al. Alteration of reproductive function but not prenatal sexual development after insertional disruption of the mouse estrogen receptor gene. *Proc Natl Acad Sci U S A* 1993; **90**: 162–6.

48. Couse JF, Korach KS. Exploring the role of sex steroids through studies of receptor deficient mice. *J Mol Med* 1998; **76**: 497–511.

49. Hess RA, Bunick D, Lee K-H et al. A role for oestrogens in the male reproductive system. *Nature* 1997; **390**: 509–12.

50. Das SK, Taylor JA, Korach KS et al. Estrogenic responses in estrogen receptor-α deficient mice reveal a distinct estrogen signaling pathway. *Proc Natl Acad Sci U S A* 1997; **94**: 12 786–91.

51. Shughrue PJ, Lubahn DB, Negro-Villar A et al. Responses in the brain of estrogen receptor α-disrupted mice. *Proc Natl Acad Sci U S A* 1997; **94**: 11 008–12.

52. Krege JH, Hodgin JB, Couse JF et al. Generation and reproductive phenotypes of mice lacking estrogen receptor β. *Proc Natl Acad Sci U S A* 1998; **95**: 15 677–82.

53. Smith EP, Boyd J, Frank GR et al. Estrogen resistance caused by a mutation in the estrogen receptor gene in a man. *N Engl J Med* 1994; **331**: 1056–61.

54. Pettersson K, Grandien K, Kuiper GGJM, Gustafsson J-Å. Mouse estrogen receptor β forms estrogen response element-binding heterodimers with estrogen receptor α. *Mol Endocrinol* 1997; **11**: 1486–96.

55. Pace P, Taylor J, Suntharalingam S et al. Human estrogen receptor β binds DNA in a manner similar to and dimerizes with estrogen receptor α. *J Biol Chem* 1997; **272**: 25 832–8.

56. Kuiper GGJM, Gustafsson J-Å. The novel estrogen receptor-β subtype: potential role in the cell- and promoter-specific actions of estrogens and anti-estrogens. *FEBS Lett* 1997; **410**: 87–90.

57. Cowley SM, Hoare S, Mosselman S, Parker MG. Estrogen receptors α and β form heterodimers on DNA. *J Biol Chem* 1997; **272**: 19 858–62.

58. Pennie WD, Aldridge TC, Brooks AN. Differential activation by xenoestrogens of ERα and ERβ when linked to different response elements. *J Endocrinol* 1998; **158**: R11–R14.

59. Hyder SM, Chiapetta C, Stancel GM. Interaction of human estrogen receptors α and β with the same naturally occurring estrogen response elements. *Biochem Pharmacol* 1999; **57**: 597–601.

60. Nilsson S, Kuiper GGJM, Gustafsson J-Å, ERβ: a novel estrogen receptor offers the potential for new drug development. *Trends Endocrinol Metab* 1998; **9**: 387–95.

61. Sun J, Meyers MJ, Fink BE et al. Novel ligands that function as selective estrogens or antiestrogens for estrogen receptor α or estrogen receptor β. *Endocrinology* 1999; **140**: 800–4.

62. Jensen EV, Jacobson HI. Basic guides to the mechanism of estrogen action. *Recent Prog Horm Res* 1962; **18**: 387–414.

63. Gorski J, Toft D, Shyamala G et al. Hormone receptors: studies on the interaction of estrogen with the uterus. *Recent Prog Horm Res* 1968; **24**: 45–81.

4

Skeletal effects of selective oestrogen receptor modulators (SERMs)

Jean-Yves Reginster, Anne-Noelle Taquet, Olivier A Bruyere

SERMs have been consistently shown to reduce bone turnover, prevent oestrogen deficiency-induced bone loss and reduce osteoporotic vertebral fractures in a similar way to oestrogens. Raloxifene, which has an oestrogen agonistic effect on bone with no stimulation of reproductive tissue, appears to be a first-line treatment strategy in the prevention and treatment of postmenopausal osteoporosis.

Introduction

Ovarian failure and subsequent oestrogen depletion are known to result in accelerated bone loss as a result of a rapid increase in osteoclast-mediated bone resorption.[1] In some animal models, oophorectomy is frequently followed by an increase in turnover of cancellous and cortical bone,[2,3] with bone resorption increasing more than bone formation, resulting in a net loss of bone mineral density. In humans, bone loss has been clearly documented as a major adverse consequence of the menopause whether occurring spontaneously, surgically or following chemotherapy or irradiation.[4–6] Hormone replacement therapy (oestrogens alone or oestrogen/progestagen combination) is often prescribed in the years following the menopause to decrease the symptoms (hot flushes, vaginal dryness) that result from decreased circulating oestrogen levels. In rats, HRT was shown to reverse ovariectomy-mediated bone loss.[7] In postmenopausal women, HRT use is associated with prevention of cancellous and cortical bone loss[8,9] and with a delay in the onset of postmenopausal osteoporosis. Reduction of spine, forearm and hip fractures in HRT-treated women is based only on epidemiological trials[10–13] and has not been documented in large prospective, randomized studies.[14, 15] However, several questions related to the time of onset, duration, dose and regimen of HRT for optimal prevention of osteoporosis remain unanswered.[16–18] Furthermore, there are a number of undesirable effects associated with chronic use of oestrogens that limit the number of patients willing to initiate the treatment and that reduce compliance.[19] The main issues perceived by women who might otherwise be candidates for HRT include an increased risk of endometrial cancer,[20] which may persist despite the addition of progestin,[21] and an increased risk of breast cancer.[22] Other less serious side-effects include resumption of menses, mastodynia and weight gain. On the other hand, HRT may also reduce coronary heart disease[23,24] (although this effect was not confirmed in a recent secondary prevention trial[14]), improve cognitive function,[25] including maintenance of short-term memory, and ameliorate the clinical symptoms of Alzheimer's disease.[26]

An ideal treatment for postmenopausal women would thus include an oestrogen-like effect on the skeleton, without production of the significant side-effects, occurring mainly in reproductive tissues.

Bone-specific agents like calcitonin, fluoride or bisphosphonates have been shown to prevent postmenopausal bone loss and, to some extent, to reduce fracture rates in established osteoporosis.[27–29] Besides some potential specific toxicity,[27–29] none of these compounds is associated with significant extraskeletal benefits for postmenopausal women. During the last decade, a new family of compounds, called 'selective oestrogen receptor modulators' (SERMs), was identified. SERMs are defined as compounds which produce oestrogen agonism in one or more desired target tissue (e.g. bone) together with oestrogen antagonism and/or minimal agonism (i.e. clinically insignificant) in reproductive tissues such as the breast or uterus.[30] We review here the current evidence of a bone-protective effect for marketed or currently developed SERMs.

Tamoxifen

Tamoxifen, a triphenylethylene, was initially developed for the treatment of breast cancer and classified as an 'antioestrogen'. Since that time, it has been widely used not only for the treatment of breast cancer,[31] where it is now considered to be standard therapy for postmenopausal women with oestrogen receptor positive and node positive cancers, but also for prophylaxis.[32] Concomitantly, oestrogen agonist effects of tamoxifen were demonstrated on serum cholesterol.[33] From randomized breast cancer trials, a significant reduction in cardiovascular diseases and mortality in tamoxifen-treated patients versus placebo was also documented.[34]

Reports on the effects of tamoxifen on bone are conflicting. While a reduction of bone mass was reported in tamoxifen-treated rats,[35,36] a large number of studies reported an antiresorptive action of tamoxifen and a preservation of bone mass in the lumbar spine and proximal femur in the same species.[37–40] There is now evidence that tamoxifen directly inhibits osteoclast activity[40] and, through a positive effect on insulin-like growth factor-1 secretion, may exert enhancing effects on bone formation.[41] In ovarian hormone-deficient rats, subcutaneous pellets of tamoxifen inhibit osteoclast-mediated resorption of cancellous bone at concentrations that are not uterotrophic (5 mg slow-release).[42] In ovariectomized rats, treated with oral tamoxifen (0.1 or 1 mg/kg per day) or ethinyloestradiol (30 μg/kg per day) for 4 weeks, loss of femoral and lumbar vertebral bone density was prevented as was the decrease in bone mass and the increase in bone resorption and bone turnover in proximal tibial metaphyses. However, at these doses, uterine weight and uterine cross-sectional tissue area exhibit an intermediate pattern between control and ethinyloestradiol-treated animals.[43] Tamoxifen was also reported partially to prevent bone loss induced by sciatic neurotomy in rats.[44] In postmenopausal women with breast cancer, oral tamoxifen (20 mg/day) significantly decreased urinary excretion cross-linked amino-terminal telopeptide of type I collagen (33%), serum osteocalcin (25%) and serum amino-terminal propeptide of type I procollagen (22%), but failed to exhibit a significant effect on the bone-specific iso-enzyme of serum alkaline phosphatase.[45] While an early report of a study performed in premenopausal women with breast cancer demonstrated a non-significant decrease in bone mineral content of distal radius (assessed by single photon absorptiometry) in placebo and tamoxifen-treated patients after 12 months,[46] several authors have reported that tamoxifen given to postmenopausal women with breast cancer preserved bone mineral density.[47–53] These effects were observed at oral doses from 20 to 40 mg/day after 1 year,[45,47] 2 years,[48,50] 5 years[52–54] and even 7 years.[55] Overall, the bone protective effect of tamoxifen was apparent after 6 months of therapy, plateaued after 1 year and remained stable until the end of follow-up. The effect of tamoxifen was predominant at the spine but there were also modest increases of bone mineral density at the hip.[56,57] The effect of tamoxifen on bone mineral density was also assessed in normal, late postmenopausal women. Subjects taking 20 mg/day of tamoxifen for 2 years showed a decrease in serum levels of alkaline phosphatase and urinary excretion of collagen N-telopeptide, an increase in bone mineral density of the lumbar spine, decreased loss of total body bone mineral density and no difference in bone mineral density of the femur when compared with those receiving a placebo.[58]

However, despite these promising results observed in the skeleton, a major concern limiting widespread use of tamoxifen in the prevention and treatment of postmenopausal osteoporosis in women without breast cancer is uterine stimulation and increased risk of endometrial cancer.[59,60]

Raloxifene

Raloxifene and its hydrochloride salt form, previously known as keoxifene, are benzothiophene derivatives that, as for tamoxifen, were initially investigated as a treatment for advanced breast cancer.[20,61] Raloxifene was also shown to inhibit the hypertrophy of the uterus in response to oestrogens[19,62] and to reduce serum cholesterol levels.[19] In the perspective of this unique pharmacological profile, raloxifene became the subject of an extensive investigational programme defined to evaluate its skeletal properties.

On a molecular basis, raloxifene activates the gene encoding transforming growth factor β (TGFβ3), which, together with other growth factors and cytokines, induces production of osteoblasts and inhibits the activity and shortens the lifespan of osteoclasts.[63,64] In vitro, raloxifene and oestrogen inhibit, with similar potency and magnitude, interleukin-6-induced differentiation and resorptive activity of mammalian osteoclasts.[65] In the human-female-derived SaOS-2 osteoblast-like cell line, raloxifene, from a concentration of 1 nmol/l, dose-dependently stimulated creatine-kinase activity, a marker of cell division.[63] Beneficial oestrogen agonist-like effects of raloxifene have been characterized extensively in ovariectomized rats. As an in vivo correlate of in vitro experiments, raloxifene and oestrogens produce parallel reductions of serum interleukin-6 levels in ovariectomized rats to levels observed in sham controls.[66] In the same model, oral administration of raloxifene (0.1–10 mg/kg per day) for 5 weeks induced similar effects (preservation of bone mineral density in the distal femur and proximal tibia) to those of 0.1 mg/kg per day orally of ethinyloestradiol.[19] Noteworthy in this experiment was the lack of significant oestrogenic effect on uterine tissue in raloxifene-treated animals. The effects of ovariectomy on 6 month old rats' spinal bone mineral density, femoral moment of inertia, dry weight and volume, and, to a lesser extent, femoral bone mineral density were similarly inhibited in an indistinguishable fashion by 17-ßoestradiol (100 µg/kg per day, subcutaneously) and raloxifene hydrochloride (1 mg/kg per day, orally), with a half-maximally effective dose of raloxifene on L1–L4 bone mineral density between 0.1 and 1.0 mg/kg per day.[67] When these animals were examined by peripheral computed tomography, the proximal tibia showed a 17% reduction in mineral density 31 days after ovariectomy with a progressive increase in the cross-sectional area of the proximal tibiae, loss of cancellous bone, widening of marrow spaces and thinning of the cortical bone wall opposite the fibula. Regression analysis of the dose-dependent protective effects of raloxifene showed half-maximal efficacy on the tibial mineral density at 0.4 mg/kg per day. By comparison, 17α-ethinyloestradiol showed dose-dependent effects with $ED_{50} = 0.013$ mg/kg per day.[68] After 6 months of oral administration, raloxifene and ethinyloestradiol produced equivalent beneficial effects on the biomechanical properties of the vertebra (load to fracture) and the femoral neck (shear to failure) compared with ovariectomized controls, with a significant correlation between vertebral strength and vertebral bone mineral density.[69]

In early postmenopausal women, randomly assigned to raloxifene, oestrogen or no treatment, both raloxifene (60 mg/day) and oestrogen (0.625 mg/day conjugated equine oestrogens) plus 5 mg medroxyprogesterone/day for the first 2 weeks of each month produced a significant positive calcium balance shift, assessed by using calcium tracer kinetic methods, for up to 31 weeks of therapy. At this timepoint resorption was reduced by both agents, though to a greater extent with oestrogens, and formation was reduced by oestrogens but not by raloxifene, so that the general pattern of bone remodelling was similarly affected by the two agents.[70] In healthy postmenopausal women, raloxifene hydrochloride (200–600 mg/day) and conjugated equine oestrogens (0.625 mg/day), given for 8 weeks, decreased to a similar extent biochemical markers of bone remodelling, i.e. serum alkaline phosphatase (range 10–11%), serum osteocalcin (range 21–26%), urinary pyridinoline cross-links (range 20–26%) and urinary calcium excretion (range 45–72%).[71] This oestrogen-agonist like effect on bone turnover translated into significant increases in bone mineral density of the lumbar spine, hip and total body when postmenopausal women, aged 45–60 years and within 2–8 years of the menopause, with T-scores for bone mineral density of the lumbar spine between −2.5 and +2.0, were randomized for 24 months to receive placebo or 30, 60 or

150 mg/day of raloxifene for 24 months. At 24 months, the mean (SE) difference in the change in bone mineral density between the women receiving 60 mg raloxifene and those receiving placebo was 2.4% (0.4%) for the lumbar spine, 2.4% (0.4%) for the total hip and 2.0% (0.4%) for the total body. A subgroup analysis demonstrated that the increases in bone mineral density in lumbar spine and hip during therapy were similar regardless of the initial bone mineral density, level of bone turnover as assessed by baseline biochemical determinations, the age, the body mass index and the history of oestrogen or thiazide therapy.[72]

Raloxifene (60 or 120 mg/day) was also administered to postmenopausal women with at least one prevalent vertebral fracture and compared in a 2-year double-blind, placebo-controlled, prospective, randomized study to a control group receiving 750 mg of calcium and 400 iu vitamin D daily. Biochemical markers of bone remodelling, i.e. serum bone-specific alkaline phosphatase [−24% (6%)], osteocalcin [−36% (6%)] and urinary C-telopeptide fragment of type I collagen/creatinine [−36% (8%)] (values for raloxifene 60 mg/day), were significantly decreased with non-significant trends towards an increase over controls in bone mineral density for lumbar spine, total body and total hip.[73] Similar results for biochemical markers of bone resorption and bone mineral density were obtained in studies involving European[74] and Asian[75] populations. In a multicentre, randomized, double-blind, placebo-controlled study designed to test the hypothesis that treatment with raloxifene reduces the risk of vertebral fractures in postmenopausal women aged up to 80 years with osteoporosis (hip or spine bone mineral density T-score < -2.5, with or without prevalent vertebral fracture), 7705 women were enrolled into two substudies based on the presence of hip or spine T-score < -2.5 ($n = 5064$, substudy I) or existing vertebral fracture ($n = 2641$, substudy II). Women were randomized to placebo, raloxifene 60 mg/day or raloxifene 120 mg/day; all were given supplemental calcium (500 mg/day) and vitamin D (400 iu/day). At 36 months in substudy I, 77 (2.5%) women treated with raloxifene (pooled doses) compared with 68 (4.5%) women treated with placebo had one or more incident vertebral fractures (relative risk 0.5; 95% confidence interval 0.4–0.8). In substudy II at 36 months, 195 (12.7%) women treated with raloxifene (pooled doses) compared with 163 (21.2%) women treated with placebo had one or more incident vertebral fracture (relative risk 0.6; 95% confidence interval 0.4–0.8). In both substudies, significant reductions in the risk of incident vertebral fracture were observed for both 60 mg and 120 mg doses of raloxifene (***Figure 4.1***).[76] There was no difference between the raloxifene (pooled doses) and placebo groups in the risk of non-traumatic, non-vertebral fracture (relative risk

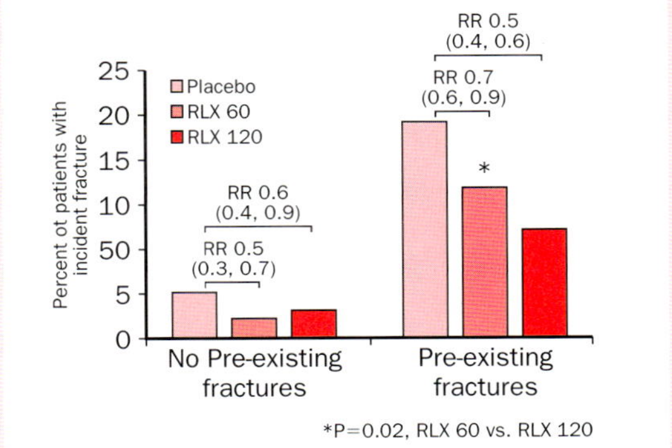

Figure 4.1
Reduction in new vertebral fractures in patients with or without pre-existing fractures. Data from reference 76.

0.9; 95% confidence interval 0.8–1.1, (pooled substudies).[76] From a cost–utility analysis, based on a Swedish database, it appears that raloxifene can be targeted cost-effectively to postmenopausal women with osteopenia with a value of 27,000 US dollars (USD) quality adjusted life year (QALY) gained in postmenopausal women aged 55 years with osteopenia (relative risk for hip fracture 2.6); and 20,400 USD/QALY gained when targeted to women aged 65 or older or at high risk (relative risk 3.0) for hip fracture.[77]

Other currently developed SERMs

Recent studies have suggested that several compounds may demonstrate a SERMs profile, including other triphenylethylenes (e.g. clomiphene, toremifene, droloxifene or idoxifene), benzothiophenes (LY117018 raloxifene analogue),[78] benzopyrans, tetrahydronaphthylenes (e.g. CP336156) and structurally distinct molecules such as levormeloxifene.[56] Of interest, a recent report suggests that one of the plant-derived oestrogenic substances, the phytoestrogen coumestrol, can be modified to act as an oestrogen agonist/antagonist.[56,79]

Relatively few data are currently available concerning the skeletal effects of these compounds. When compared with tamoxifen in postmenopausal women with breast cancer, toremifene (40 mg/day) prevented the age related decrease in bone mineral density but failed to influence bone turnover markers or to increase bone mineral density at any site.[45]

Droloxifene (1.0 mg/kg per os daily)

prevented loss of femoral and lumbar vertebral bone mineral density in 5-month-old ovariectomized rats.[80] When compared with other inhibitors of bone resorption, droloxifene acted similarly to tamoxifen (0.1 and 1 mg/kg per day) or ethinyloestradiol (30 μg/kg per day), but with a lack of significant oestrogenic effects on uterine tissue.[43] Similar findings were obtained when comparing oestradiol (30 μg/kg per day, subcutaneously) or oral droloxifene (2.5, 5 or 10 mg/kg per day) for 8 weeks in 19-month-old ovariectomized rats. In this experiment, droloxifene, at all doses, prevented the decrease in bone mineral density of the distal femoral metaphysis induced by ovariectomy and, at the dose of 10 mg/kg per day, also prevented the decrease in bone mineral density observed in the whole femora, femoral shaft and proximal femora.[81]

Raloxifene analogue (LY 117018HCl) (3 mg/kg per day per os) was given for 28 days to cyclosporin-A treated ovariectomized rats. In this model LY 117018 completely prevented the high turnover osteopenia caused by oophorectomy and was able to attenuate substantially the effects of cyclosporin-A in ovariectomized rats.[82]

In a preliminary report, CP336156, given alone for 5.5 months to ovariectomized 3.5-month-old rats (0.1 mg/kg per day) significantly increased total femoral bone area, bone mineral content and density while its combination with CP424391, an orally active growth hormone secretagogue, resulted in further increases.[83] The same compound (0.1 mg/kg per day for 60 days), combined with the 1-34 parathyroid hormone fragments (40 μg/kg per day subcutaneously) significantly increased the cancellous volume (+24%) of proximal tibia and the initial maximum load of distal femora (+86%) decreasing bone resorption more than bone formation when compared with parathyroid hormone alone, thus supporting a strategy for combining SERMs and anabolic agents for the treatment of established osteoporosis.[84]

Idoxifene (5–10 mg/day per os) showed a reduction in bone turnover in a 3-month dose-ranging study and, in an open label extension (5 mg/day) after 12–15 months of therapy, an increase in lumbar bone mineral density (+1.73%) was documented.[85]

For all these compounds, further development in accordance with guidelines for the registration of drugs to be used in the prevention and treatment of involutional osteoporosis in women[86] will be requested before evaluation of their risk:benefit ratio in daily practice.

References

1. Richelson LS, Wahner HW, Melton LJ III et al. Relative contribution of aging and estrogen deficiency to postmenopausal bone loss. *N Engl J Med* 1984; **311**: 1273–5.

2. Wronski TJ, Dann LM, Scott KS, Cintron M. Long-term effects of ovariectomy and aging

on the rat skeleton. *Calcif Tissue Int* 1989; **45**: 360–6.

3. Kalu DN. The ovariectomized rat model of postmenopausal bone loss. *Bone Miner* 1991; **15**: 175–92.
4. Riggs BL, Melton LJ III. Involutional osteoporosis. *N Engl J Med* 1986; **314**: 1676–86.
5. Aitken JM, Hart DM, Anderson JB et al. Osteoporosis after oophorectomy for non-malignant disease in premenopausal women. *Br Med J* 1973; **2**: 325–8.
6. Bruning PF, de Jong-Bakker M, van den Ende A et al. Bone mineral density after adjuvant chemotherapy for premenopausal breast cancer. *Br J Cancer* 1990; **61**: 308–10.
7. Wronski TJ, Cintron M, Doherty AL, Dann LM. Estrogen treatment prevents osteopenia and depresses bone turnover in ovariectomized rats. *Endocrinology* 1988; **123**: 681–6.
8. Lindsay R, Hart DM, Forrest C, Baird C. Prevention of spinal osteoporosis in oophorectomised women. *Lancet* 1980; **i**: 1151–4.
9. Christiansen C, Christensen MS, McNair P et al. Prevention of early postmenopausal bone loss: controlled 2-year study in 315 normal females. *Eur J Clin Invest* 1980; **10**: 273–9.
10. Cauley JA, Seeley DG, Ensrud K et al. Estrogen replacement therapy and fractures in older women. *Ann Intern Med* 1995; **122**: 9–16.
11. Naessen T, Persson I, Adami HO et al. Hormone replacement therapy and the risk for hip fracture. A prospective, population-based cohort study. *Ann Intern Med* 1990; **113**: 95–103.
12. Weiss NS, Ure CL, Ballard JH et al. Decreased risk of fractures of the hip and lower forearm with postmenopausal use of estrogen. *N Engl J Med* 1980; **303**: 1195–8.
13. Kanis JA, Johnell O, Gullberg B et al. Evidence for efficacy of drugs affecting bone metabolism in preventing hip fracture. *Br Med J* 1992; **305**: 1124–8.
14. Hulley SH, Grady D, Bush T et al. Randomized trial of estrogen plus progestin for secondary prevention of coronary heart disease in postmenopausal women. *JAMA* 1998; **280**: 605–13.
15. Compston JE. HRT and osteoporosis. *Br Med Bull* 1992; **48**: 309–44.
16. Reginster JY, Sarlet N, Deroisy R et al. Minimal levels of estradiol preventing postmenopausal bone loss. *Calcif Tissue Int* 1992; **51**: 340–3
17. Quigley ME, Martin PL, Burnier AM, Brooks P. Estrogen therapy arrests bone loss in elderly women. *Am J Obstet Gynecol* 1987; **156**: 1516–23.
18. Felson DT, Zhang Y, Hannan MT et al. The effect of postmenopausal estrogen therapy on bone density in elderly women. *N Engl J Med* 1993; **329**: 1141–6.
19. Black LJ, Sato M, Rowley ER et al. Raloxifene (LY139481) prevents bone loss and reduces serum cholesterol without causing uterine hypertrophy in ovariectomized rats. *J Clin Invest* 1994; **93**: 63–9.
20. Grady D, Gebretsadik T, Kerlikowske K et al. Hormone replacement therapy and endometrial cancer risk: a meta-analysis. *Obstet Gynecol* 1995; **85**: 304–13.
21. Beresford SA, Weiss NS, Voigt LF, McKnight B. Risk of endometrial cancer in relation to use of oestrogen combined with cyclic progestagen therapy in postmenopausal women. *Lancet* 1997; **349**: 458–61.

22. Colditz GA, Hankinson SE, Hunter DJ et al. The use of estrogens and progestins and the risk of breast cancer in postmenopausal women. *N Engl J Med* 1995; **332**: 1589–93.

23. Barrett-Connor E, Bush TL. Estrogen and coronary heart disease in women. *JAMA* 1991; **265**: 1861–7.

24. Stampfer MJ, Colditz GA. Estrogen replacement therapy and coronary disease: a quantitative assessment of the epidemiological evidence. *Prev Med* 1991; **20**: 47–63.

25. Sherwin BB. Estrogen and/or androgen replacement therapy and cognitive functioning in surgically menopausal women. *Psychoneuroendocrinology* 1988; **13**: 345–57.

26. Honjo H, Tanaka H, Kashiwagi T et al. Senile dementia Alzheimer's type and estrogen. *Hormone Metab Res* 1995; **27**: 204–7.

27. Reginster JY. Calcitonin for prevention and treatment of osteoporosis. *Am J Med* 1993; **95**: 44–7.

28. Reginster JY, Paul I, Gosset C. Current status of fluoride salts to treat postmenopausal osteoporosis. *Curr Opin Orthop* 1998; **9**: 7–10.

29. Reginster JY, Gosset C, Fraikin G. Bisphosphonates for the treatment of osteoporosis. In: Meunier PJ (ed). *Osteoporosis: Diagnosis and Management.* Martin Dunitz Publishers: London, 1998: 123–30

30. Kauffman RF, Bryant HU. Effective therapeutic management of the postmenopausal state will be a cornerstone in strategies for preserving or improving women's health in the 21st century. Selective estrogen receptor modulators. *Drugs News & Perspectives* 1995; **8**: 531–9.

31. Early Breast Cancer Trialists' Collaborative Group. Systemic treatment of early breast cancer by hormonal, cytotoxic, or immune therapy. *Lancet* 1992; **339**: 71–85.

32. Powles TJ. The case for clinical trials of tamoxifen for prevention of breast cancer. *Lancet* 1992; **340**: 1145–7.

33. Sismondi P, Biglia N, Giai M et al. Metabolic effects of tamoxifen in postmenopause. *Anticancer Res* 1994; **14**: 2237–44.

34. Rutqvist LE, Mattson A. Cardiac and thromboembolic morbidity among postmenopausal women with early stage breast cancer in randomized trial of adjuvant tamoxifen. *J Natl Cancer Inst* 1993; **85**: 1398–406.

35. Parvizi ST, Minnie HW, Bauss F, Ziegler R. Antioestrogen treatment produces loss of bone mass as a side effect in the rat. *Acta Endocrinol* 1985; **108**: 168–71.

36. Feldmann S, Minne HW, Parvizi S et al. Antioestrogen and antiandrogen administration reduce bone mass in the rat. *Bone Miner* 1989; **7**: 245–54.

37. Kalu DN, Salerno E, Liu CC et al. A comparative study of the actions of tamoxifen, estrogen and progesterone in the ovariectomized rat. *Bone Miner* 1991; **15**: 109–24.

38. Moon LY, Wakley GK, Turner RT. Dose-dependent effects of tamoxifen on long bones of growing rats: influence of ovarian status. *Endocrinology* 1991; **129**: 1568–74.

39. Turner RT, Wakley GK, Hannon KS, Bell NH. Tamoxifen prevents the skeletal effects of ovarian hormone deficiency in rats. *J Bone Miner Res* 1987; **2**: 449–56.

40. Stewart PJ, Stern PH. Effects of the antiestrogens tamoxifen and clomiphene on bone resorption in vitro. *Endocrinology* 1986; **118**: 125–31.

41. Colletti RB, Roberts JD, Devlin JT, Copeland KC. Effects of tamoxifen on plasma insulin-like growth factor I in patients with breast cancer. *Cancer Res* 1989; **49**: 1882–4.

42. Turner RT, Wakley GK, Hannon KS, Bell NH. Tamoxifen inhibits osteoclast-mediated resorption of trabecular bone in ovarian hormone-deficient rats. *Endocrinology* 1988; **122**: 1146–50.

43. Ke HZ, Chen HK, Simmons HA et al. Comparative effects of droloxifene, tamoxifen and estrogen on bone, serum cholesterol, and uterine histology in the ovariectomized rat model. *Bone* 1997; **20**: 31–9.

44. Wakley GK, Baum BL, Hannon KS, Turner RT. The effects of tamoxifen on the osteopenia induced by sciatic neurotomy in the rat: a histomorphometric study. *Calcif Tissue Int* 1988; **43**: 383–8.

45. Marttunen MB, Hietanen P, Titinen A, Ylikorkala O. Comparison of effects of tamoxifen and toremifene on bone biochemistry and bone mineral density in postmenopausal breast cancer patients. *J Clin Endocrinol Metab* 1998; **83**: 1158–62.

46. Gotfredsen A, Christiansen C, Palshof T. The effect of tamoxifen on bone mineral content in premenopausal women with breast cancer. *Cancer* 1984; **53**: 853–7.

47. Turken S, Siris E, Seldin D et al. Effects of tamoxifen on spinal bone density in women with breast cancer. *J Natl Cancer Inst* 1989; **81**: 1086–8.

48. Kristensen B, Ejlertsen B, Dalgaard P et al. Tamoxifen and bone metabolism in postmenopausal low-risk breast cancer patients: a randomized study. *J Clin Oncol* 1994; **12**: 992–7.

49. Wright CD, Garrahan NJ, Stanton M et al. Effect of long-term tamoxifen therapy on cancellous bone remodeling and structure in women with breast cancer. *J Bone Miner Res* 1994; **9**: 153–9.

50. Love RR, Mazess RB, Tormey DC et al. Bone mineral density in women with breast cancer treated with adjuvant tamoxifen for at least two years. *Breast Cancer Res Treat* 1988; **12**: 297–301.

51. Love RR, Mazess RB, Barden HS et al. Effects of tamoxifen on bone mineral density in postmenopausal women with breast cancer. *N Engl J Med* 1992; **326**: 852–6.

52. Neal AJ, Evans K, Hoskin PJ. Does long-term administration of tamoxifen affect bone mineral density. *Eur J Cancer* 1993; **29A**: 1971–3.

53. Love RR, Barden HS, Mazess RB et al. Effect of tamoxifen on lumbar spine bone mineral density in postmenopausal women after 5 years. *Arch Intern Med* 1994; **154**: 2585–8.

54. Powles TJ, Hickish T, Kanis JA et al. Effect of tamoxifen on bone mineral density measured by dual-energy X-ray absorptiometry in healthy premenopausal and postmenopausal women. *J Clin Oncol* 1996; **14**: 78–84.

55. Fornander RT, Rutqvist LE, Sjörberg HE et al. Long-term adjuvant tamoxifen in early breast cancer: effect on bone mineral density in postmenopausal women. *J Clin Oncol* 1990; **8**: 1019–24.

56. Mitlak BH, Cohen FJ. In search of optimal long-term female hormone replacement: the potential of selective estrogen receptor modulators. *Horm Res* 1997; **48**: 155–63.

57. Chang J, Powles TJ, Ashley SE et al. The effect of tamoxifen and hormone replacement therapy on serum cholesterol, bone mineral density and coagulation factors in healthy postmenopausal women participating in a randomized, controlled tamoxifen prevention study. *Ann Oncol* 1996; 7: 671–5.

58. Grey AB, Stapleton JP, Evans MC et al. The effect of the antiestrogen tamoxifen on bone mineral density in normal late postmenopausal women. *Am J Med* 1995; **99**: 636–41.

59. Fisher B, Constantino JP, Redmond CK et al. Endometrial cancer in tamoxifen-treated breast cancer patients: findings from the National Surgical Adjuvant Breast and Bowel Project. *J Natl Cancer Inst* 1994; **86**: 527–37.

60. Ross D, Whitehead M. Hormonal manipulation and gynecological cancer: the tamoxifen dilemma. *Curr Opin Obstet Gynecol* 1995; 7: 63–8.

61. Hol T, Cox MB, Bryant HU, Draper MW. Selective estrogen receptor modulators and postmenopausal women's health. *J Women's Health* 1997; **6**: 523–30.

62. Black LJ, Jones CD, Facone JR. Antagonism of estrogen action with a new benzothiophene derived antiestrogen. *Life Sci* 1993; **32**: 1031–6.

63. Balfour JA, Goa KL. Raloxifene. *Drugs Aging* 1998; **12**: 335–42.

64. Yang NN, Bryant HU, Hardikar S et al. Estrogen and raloxifene stimulate transforming growth factor-beta 3 gene expression in rat bone: apotentiazl mechanism for estrogen- or raloxifene-mediated bone maintenance. *Endocrinology* 1996; **137**: 2075–84.

65. Sato M, Rippy MK, Bryant HU. Raloxifene, tamoxifen, nafoxidine or estrogen effects on reproductive and non-reproductive tissues in ovariectomized rats. *FASEB J* 1996; **10**: 905–12.

66. Glasebrook AL, Short LL, Cole HW et al. Regulation of serum IL-6 by raloxifene in an ovariectomized rat model. *Bone* 1995; **16**: 99.

67. Sato M, McClintock C, Kim J et al. Dual-energy X-ray absorptiometry of raloxifene effects on the lumbar vertebrae and femora of ovariectomized rats. *J Bone Miner Res* 1994; **9**: 715–24.

68. Sato M, Kim J, Short LL et al. Longitudinal and cross-sectional analysis of raloxifene effects on tibiae from ovariectomized aged rats. *J Pharmacol Exp Ther* 1995; **272**: 1252–9.

69. Turner CH, Sato M, Bryant HU. Raloxifene preserves bone strength and bone mass in ovariectomized rats. *Endocrinology* 1994; **135**: 2001–5.

70. Heaney RP, Draper MW. Raloxifene and estrogen: comparative bone-remodeling kinetics. *J Clin Endocrinol Metab* 1997; **82**: 3425–9.

71. Draper MW, Flowers DE, Huster WJ et al. A controlled trial of raloxifene (LY139481) HCl: impact on bone turnover and serum lipid profile in healthy postmenopausal women. *J Bone Miner Res* 1996; **11**: 835–42.

72. Delmas PD, Bjarnason NH, Mitlak BH et al. Effects of raloxifene on bone mineral density, serum cholesterol concentrations, and uterine endometrium in postmenopausal women. *N Engl J Med* 1997; **337**: 1641–7.

73. Lufkin EG, Whitaker MD, Nickelsen T et al. Treatment of established postmenopausal osteoporosis with raloxifene: a randomized trial. *J Bone Miner Res* 1998; **13**: 1747–54.

74. Meunier PJ, Vignot E, Garnero P et al. Postmenopausal women with osteoporosis: effects of raloxifene on bone mineral density in the hip and lumbar spine. *Bone* 1998; **23**: S295.

75. Morii H, Fujita T, Ishii J et al. Raloxifene for treatment of osteoporosis: determination of an

adequate dose in Japanese women. *Bone* 1998; **23**: S610.

76. Ettinger B, Black DM, Mitlak BH et al. Reduction of vertebral fracture risk in postmenopausal women with osteoporosis treated with raloxifene: results from a 3-year randomized clinical trial. *JAMA* 1999; **282**(7): 637–45.

77. Kanis JA, Jonnson B, Dawson A et al. Cost-effectiveness of raloxifene: an economic evaluation based on Swedish data. *Bone* 1998; **23**: W398.

78. Bryant HU, Glasebrook AL, Yang NN, Sato M. A pharmacological review of raloxifene. *J Bone Miner Metab* 1996; **14**: 1–9.

79. Grese TA, Cole HW, Magee DE et al. Conversion of the phytoestrogen coumestrol into a selective estrogen receptor modulator (SERM) by attachment of an amine-containing sidechain. *Bioorg Med Chem Lett* 1996; **6**: 2683–6.

80. Ke HZ, Simmons HA, Pirie CM et al. Droloxifene, a new estrogen antagonist/agonist, prevents bone loss in ovariectomized rats. *Endocrinology* 1995; **136**: 2435–41.

81. Chen HK, Ke HZ, Jee WSS et al. Droloxifene prevents ovariectomy-induced bone loss in tibiae and femora of aged female rats: a dual-energy X-ray absorptiometric and histomorphometric study. *J Bone Miner Res* 1995; **10**: 1256–62.

82. Bowman AR, Sass DA, Marshall I et al. Raloxifen analog (LY117018HCL) ameliorates cyclosporin A-induced osteopenia in oophorectomized rats. *J Bone Miner Res* 1996; **11**: 1191–8.

83. Ke HZ, Li M, Pan LC et al. Combined administration of a growth hormone secretagogue (GHS) and a new selective estrogen receptor modulator (SERM) increases bone and muscle mass and decreases total serum cholesterol in ovariectomized rats. *Bone* 1998; **23**: S390.

84. Ke HZ, Chidsey-Frink KL, Simmons HA et al. CP-336,156, a new selective estrogen receptor modulator (SERM), enhances the effects of parathyroid hormone in restoring bonemass and strength in ovariectomized rats. *Bone* 1998; **23**: F360.

85. Chesnut C, Weiss S, Mulder H et al. Idoxifene increases bone mineral density in osteopenic postmenopausal women. *Bone* 1998; **23**: W397.

86. Reginster JY, Compston JE, Jones EA et al. Recommendations for the registration of new chemical entities used in the prevention and treatment of osteoporosis. *Calcif Tissue Int* 1995; **57**: 247–50.

5

Effects of SERMs on the cardiovascular system

Peter Collins

SERMs reduce total and LDL cholesterol as well as lipoprotein(a) but there is no change in HDL cholesterol. Raloxifene increases HDL_2 cholesterol but there is no change in HDL cholesterol, triglycerides or plasminogen activator inhibitor (PAI-1).

Introduction

Selective oestrogen receptor modulators (SERMs) have been developed to avoid the potential harmful effects of oestrogen on a number of tissues, including the breast and uterus. They appear to share the beneficial effects of oestrogen on bone and lipids, but are not associated with an increased risk of breast or uterine carcinoma. Oestrogen relaxes coronary arteries and has long-term protective effects on the vascular system. The possibility of a beneficial effect of SERMs on the cardiovascular system is intriguing. SERMs such as raloxifene affect both the α and β oestrogen receptor (ER), which may be important in its vascular actions.[1]

It is hoped that SERMs may significantly contribute to

the improvement of women's health.[2] Emerging evidence suggests that the newer SERMs may have effects on the cardiovascular and other systems which contribute to an improvement in vascular health and function. Research over the next 5–10 years will hopefully provide definitive data on whether these newer SERMs will be able to provide cardioprotection in postmenopausal women. This brief review will outline a number of the potential beneficial effects of SERMs on the cardiovascular system.

Oestrogen

As an introduction to the potential cardiovascular effects of SERMs, a brief overview of the vascular effects of oestrogen will be given. Present evidence suggests that the risk of coronary heart disease and oesteoporosis in postmenopausal women is reduced if they are current users of hormone replacement therapy (HRT).[3,4] Favourable effects of oestrogen on plasma lipids have clearly and consistently been shown.[5] Oestrogen also has direct relaxing properties on blood vessels, including coronary arteries from animals and humans in vivo.[6–8] A combination of these mechanisms may contribute to protection against atheroma development and to arterial health.[9]

In rabbit coronary artery rings, acute oestrogen-induced relaxation has been shown to be endothelium-independent.[6] Rings without endothelium relax to a similar degree as rings with endothelium, and inhibition of nitric oxide synthase did not alter the relaxation response.[6] Calcium antagonism at the level of the coronary myocyte was shown to be a mechanism of relaxation by oestrogen.[10] This effect of oestrogen was not dependent on the classical ER.[7] Studies have also shown an enhancement of endothelium-dependent responses in a variety of vessels.[11–15]

Chronic exposure to oestrogen can result in an increase in the release of nitric oxide (NO) from the vascular endothelium.[13,16–18] This effect is ER-dependent,[18] supported by the identification of the ER in human coronary endothelial cells.[19] Oestrogen therefore has both receptor- and non-receptor-dependent effects on blood vessels which contribute to its vasorelaxing properties and possibly its long-term cardioprotective effects.

Effects of SERMs on the cardiovascular system

Effects of SERMs on serum lipids

Studies have shown a benefit of oestrogen replacement therapy on serum lipids. Serum low-density lipoprotein cholesterol (LDL-C) is consistently decreased by both oral and transdermal oestrogen. Studies investigating the effects of SERMs on serum lipids and lipoproteins have demonstrated similar effects in both patients with breast cancer and healthy women. The SERM tamoxifen reduces total LDL cholesterol and lipoprotein (a).[20,21] Effects on high-density lipoprotein (HDL) are less clear and studies have shown that tamoxifen has small effects on the HDL level or no demonstrable effect.[21,22] In healthy postmenopausal women, raloxifene has been shown to change plasma lipid levels beneficially after 3 and 6 months of treatment.[23] Raloxifene significantly decreased LDL-C by 12%, which is similar to most studies with HRT. Raloxifene increased HDL_2 cholesterol by approximately 15%; this fraction is felt to be important in coronary heart disease protection in women. On the other hand, raloxifene did not significantly change HDL cholesterol, triglycerides or plasminogen activator inhibitor (PAI-1), which differs from results found with HRT. Similar findings on plasma lipids were found in a larger study investigating over 600 postmenopausal women.[24] Therefore, the effect of raloxifene on the plasma lipid profile shows consistency. These changes in lipid profile may be clinically favourable with regard to the effects on incidence of cardiovascular disease.[25,26]

SERMs and myocardial infarction

Data from randomized breast cancer clinical trials suggest that tamoxifen may be of benefit in protecting women from myocardial infarction. There are three adjuvant trials which show a reduction of cardiac morbidity in patients with low risk of death from breast cancer when treated with tamoxifen.[27–29]

The Rutqvist study had a median follow-up of 6 years. Tamoxifen therapy resulted in a statistically significant reduction in the incidence of hospital admissions due to cardiac disease; the relative hazard was 0.68 (CI 0.48–0.97, $p < 0.03$).[27] There was no difference in the tamoxifen control groups in terms of admissions due to thromboembolic disease.

In the McDonald study, 1312 women were randomized to tamoxifen or placebo.[28] Risks of myocardial infarction, other cardiac events and cerebrovascular disease were compared among non-users, former users and current users of tamoxifen. Tamoxifen use was associated with lower rates of myocardial infarction. The hazard ratio for women in the control group compared with women allocated to adjuvant therapy was 1.92 (CI 0.99–3.73). The association was more powerful for current users, suggesting that the protective effect would be lost on cessation of the therapy.

A more recent study[29] reviewed deaths occurring among women who were randomly assigned to 5 years of either tamoxifen or placebo in the B-14 trial. Three categories of heart disease were defined including: (1) deaths from a definite fatal myocardial infarction; (2) deaths from definite fatal coronary heart disease/possible myocardial infarction; and (3) deaths from possible fatal coronary heart disease. The annual death rate from coronary heart disease was lower for patients who received tamoxifen than for those who received placebo. The relative hazard of death from definite heart disease was 0.66 (CI 0.27–1.61) whereas the corresponding death rate of those receiving placebo was 0.85 (CI 0.46–1.58). The findings from this study are consistent with previous studies, suggesting that tamoxifen treatment reduces coronary heart disease among patients with breast cancer.

No such data are available for SERMs; these are awaited from larger studies. With regard to raloxifene, the recent MORE[30] study findings have shown that raloxifene increases the risk of venous thromboembolic disease in a similar way to oestrogen (relative risk 3.1; 95% CI 1.5–6.2), but it did not increase the risk of endometrial cancer.

Cardiovascular endpoint study–RUTH (raloxifene use and the heart) study

The ongoing RUTH study will test whether raloxifene HCl (60 mg/day) compared with placebo will reduce the combined endpoint of non-fatal myocardial infarction and coronary heart disease death (primary outcome) in postmenopausal women at higher risk of cardiac events.[31] Secondary endpoints will include cardiovascular death, myocardial revascularization, stroke, coronary death, all-cause mortality, hospitalization for unstable angina, all-cause hospitalization, non-coronary arterial revascularization, breast cancer, fractures and venous thrombotic events.

RUTH is an international, multicentre, double-blind, placebo-controlled, randomized, parallel clinical trial, and a total of 10 000 women will be enrolled. It is a time-to-event trial with a projected minimum follow-up of 5 years. As the largest study ever carried out in this group of women it will recruit from 26 countries and will be a mix of primary and secondary prevention patients. The RUTH trial will provide unique information on the potential benefit of this therapy in diverse medical settings and populations. Its results are eagerly awaited.

Effects of droloxifene on vascular reactivity

There are few data on the effect of SERMs on the human vasculature. One report has shown a beneficial effect of droloxifene on brachial flow-mediated dilatation in 24 postmenopausal women treated with 0.625 mg daily of continuous equine oestrogen or 60 mg per day droloxifene for 6 weeks with a 4-week washout. Droloxifene and oestrogen resulted in 37% and 27% improvements in vasodilator responses, respectively. There was no difference between oestrogen and droloxifene responses. This study suggests that droloxifene has effects on endothelial function that are similar to those of oestrogen.

Basic animal studies on raloxifene

Raloxifene and atherosclerosis

Two conflicting reports have been published on the effect of raloxifene on atherosclerosis. In one, surgically ovariectomized cynomolgus monkeys were fed an atherogenic diet and randomized to placebo, raloxifene (1 mg per kg/day), raloxifene (5 mg per kg/day), or continuous equine oestrogens.[32] The effects of raloxifene on plasma lipids in these animals were comparable to those found in postmenopausal women treated with raloxifene: a reduction in LDL cholesterol and no significant effects on HDL cholesterol. There was no evidence that raloxifene had an oestrogen agonist effect on coronary arteries. Treatment with continuous equine oestrogen resulted in a 70% reduction in coronary artery plaques relative to placebo.

This is in direct contrast with a study on the effects of raloxifene on 75 ovariectomized sexually mature female rabbits.[33] Atherosclerosis was induced by feeding the rabbits a cholesterol rich diet. After 45 weeks of therapy the raloxifene group had two-thirds of the aortic atherosclerosis (evidenced by the cholesterol content of the proximal inner part of the aorta) found in the placebo group. An oestrogen-treated group had one-third of the aortic atherosclerosis of the placebo group. These effects were only partly explained by changes in serum lipids and lipoprotein, and treatment with both oestrogen and raloxifene independently predicted the response with regard to aortic cholesterol content. These findings indicated that raloxifene potentially had an anti-atherosclerotic effect analagous to that observed with oestrogen in the rabbit model. A number of possible mechanisms may contribute to this decrease in cholesterol content in rabbits. There may be an ER-dependent effect, although this was not proved by this study. However, as pointed out in the study, the effect could only partially be explained by changes in serum lipids and lipoproteins because treatment with both oestrogen and raloxifene predicted the response of atherosclerosis independently of these variables.

Effects of raloxifene on vascular reactivity in vitro

Rat aorta

Basic animal studies support the case that raloxifene may have beneficial cardiovascular actions. As well as data from large clinical trials on tamoxifen, there are studies on raloxifene which show potential cardiovascular benefits. Raloxifene was shown to cause increased release of nitric oxide in rings of rat aorta studied in physiological experiments.[34] This study investigated the dilator responses to acetylcholine in phenylephrine-contracted aorta. It showed that these were increased by raloxifene and that this effect could be inhibited by the nitric oxide synthase inhibitor L-NAME. These data support the fact that in ovariectomized rats raloxifene enhances cholinergic, endothelium-dependent vasodilatation of the aorta. This is via stimulation of nitric oxide synthase because it was inhibited by nitric oxide synthase inhibition.

Cynomolgus monkey coronary artery

Contrasting data have been provided in the cynomolgus monkey model of atherosclerotic epicardial coronary arteries. The monkeys were fed for a 34-month period with continuous equine oestrogen, tamoxifen or control. Quantitative coronary angiography was used to measure dilator responses to intracoronary infusions of acetylcholine and nitroglycerine. Coronary arteries in the tamoxifen-treated group constricted in response to high doses of acetylcholine whereas those in the continuous equine oestrogen group did not. It was therefore concluded in this study that tamoxifen primarily had oestrogen antagonistic effects on epicardial coronary artery dilator responses in these monkeys.

Rabbit and human coronary artery

The effects of raloxifene on coronary artery vasoreactivity in vitro have been investigated.[35] Raloxifene induced significant dose-dependent relaxation of coronary arterial rings with endothelium (*Figures 5.1 and 5.2*). Relaxation occurred in rings without endothelium; however, relaxation in rings without endothelium was significantly less than in rings with endothelium. To compare the responses, 17β-oestradiol induced significant dose-dependent relaxation of coronary arterial rings with and without endothelium. Unlike the effect of raloxifene, there was no difference in the relaxation in rings with or without endothelium. The time-course of the relaxation response was longer for raloxifene than for 17β-oestradiol; relaxation curves were performed over approximately 90 minutes, whereas similar relaxation occurred over 10–15 minutes with oestrogen (*Figure 5.3*).

Incubation of the rings with an inhibitor of nitric oxide synthase inhibited raloxifene-induced relaxation in rabbit coronary arterial rings with endothelium. There was no significant difference between rings with endothelium, incubated in L-NAME, compared with endothelium-denuded rings. In rings without endothelium, incubation in raloxifene (−6.5 and −6 [log *M*]) shifted the calcium concentration-dependent contraction curves in high K^+ (80 mM) depolarization medium to the right compared with controls. Maximal contraction was also reduced (*Figure 5.4*). This shift was not reversed by incubation in the non-specific potassium channel inhibitor barium chloride.

This study demonstrated that raloxifene induced relaxation in precontracted male and female rabbit epicardial coronary arteries, with and without endothelium. The relaxation was

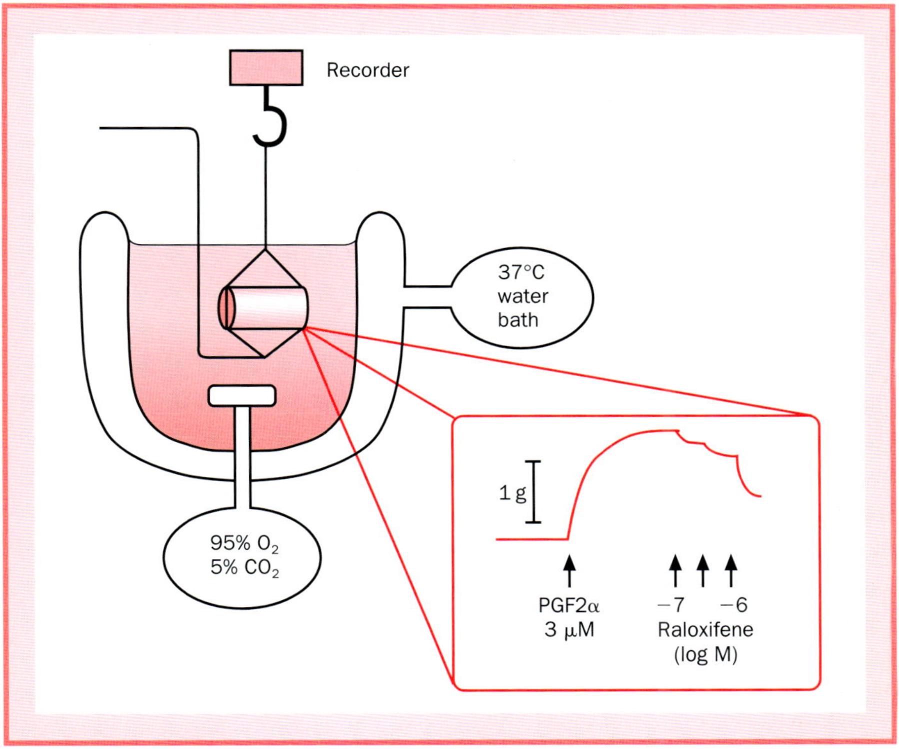

Figure 5.1
Measurement of isometric tension. Isometric tension is measured by a force transducer and recorded over time. Arterial rings are precontracted with $PGF_{2\alpha}$ before the addition of raloxifene.

significantly greater in rings with endothelium compared with rings without endothelium. This effect contrasts with that of oestrogen in this model, which did not show an endothelium-dependent relaxing effect. The raloxifene-induced relaxation was inhibited in endothelium-intact rings by L-NAME, ICI 182, 780 and barium chloride. Raloxifene shifted the calcium concentration-dependent contraction curve to the right in endothelium-denuded rings, indicating a calcium antagonistic effect. The endothelium-dependent contribution to relaxation was greatest at lower concentrations of raloxifene

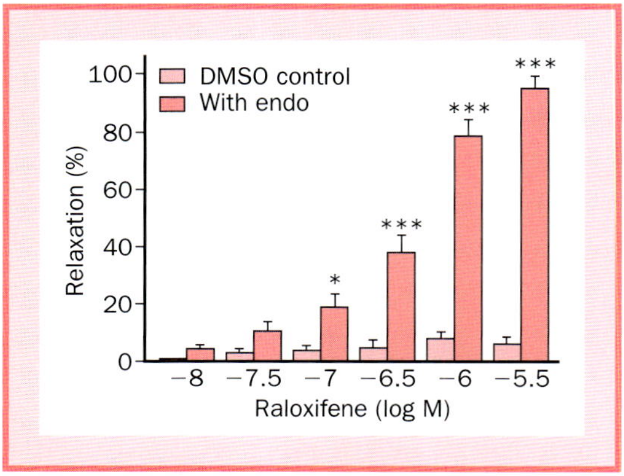

Figure 5.2
*Bar graph to show the relaxing effect of raloxifene (−8 to −5.5 [log M]) on rabbit coronary artery rings with endothelium (with endo) precontracted with prostaglandin $F_{2\alpha}$ ($PGF_{2\alpha}$ 3×10^{-6} M). Data are expressed as percentage relaxation of contraction induced by $PGF_{2\alpha}$ (mean ± SEM). Control indicates time-matched DMSO solvent controls. n = 11 − 13. *indicates significant differences in comparison with control; *$p < 0.05$; ***$p < 0.001$.*

(−6.5 and −6 [log *M*]). As the concentration of raloxifene was increased, relaxation occurred by a combined effect on the endothelium and smooth muscle. Endothelium-denuded arterial rings relaxed to approximately 100% at greater concentrations by a direct effect of raloxifene on the vascular smooth muscle myocyte.

NO is synthesized in the endothelium from L-arginine by NO synthase,[36] and can diffuse rapidly to smooth muscle, causing relaxation via stimulation of soluble guanylate cyclase and a subsequent increase in cGMP.[37] By blocking NO synthesis with L-NAME, the relaxation response to raloxifene occurs between rings with and without endothelium, implying that the endothelial contribution to raloxifene-induced relaxation is dependent on NO.

The specific ER antagonist ICI 182, 780 also inhibited raloxifene-induced relaxation in rings with endothelium, again to a level identical to relaxation in rings without endothelium. ICI 182, 780 had no effect on raloxifene-induced relaxation in coronary artery rings denuded of endothelium, suggesting that the classical ER mediates endothelium-dependent but not endothelium-independent relaxation. Raloxifene appears to interact with the ER and may increase the expression of NOS, thereby increasing endothelium-derived NO production. We were unable to distinguish between an effect on the classical ERα and the newly discovered ERβ; a recent study of oestrogen may, however, provide an explanation of the mechanism of this response.[38] Oestrogen has been shown to cause an acute (5 minutes) activation of NOS in cultured ovine

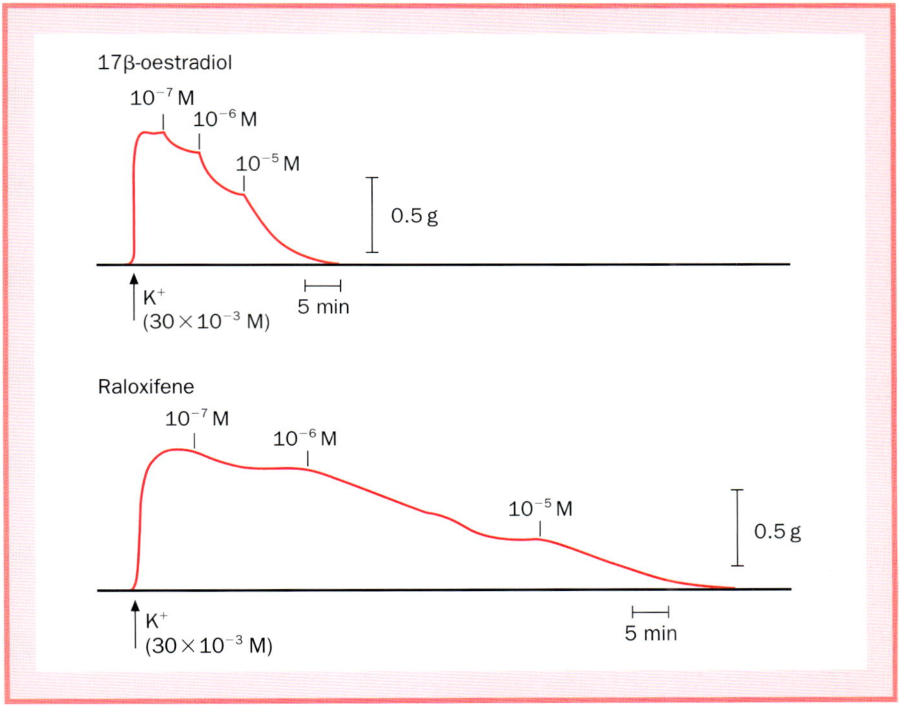

Figure 5.3
Original tracings to demonstrate the time-course of relaxation in K^+-contracted coronary arterial rings to 17β-oestradiol (10^{-7} – 10^{-5} M, top tracing) and raloxifene (10^{-7} – 10^{-5} M, bottom tracing) in rings with endothelium. Redrawn from figure originally published in Figtree et al.[35]

endothelial cells and this was unaffected by the gene transcription inhibitor actinomycin D. In an identical way to our study the NO response was inhibited by blockade of the ERα by ICI 182, 780. The inhibition of mitogen-activated protein (MAP) kinase also prevented the activation of NOS by oestrogen. Thus, the short-term activation of oestrogen is mediated by the ERα acting in a non-genomic manner. We propose that raloxifene may be working in a similar manner.

Potential-sensitive calcium channels are activated by depolarization of the plasma

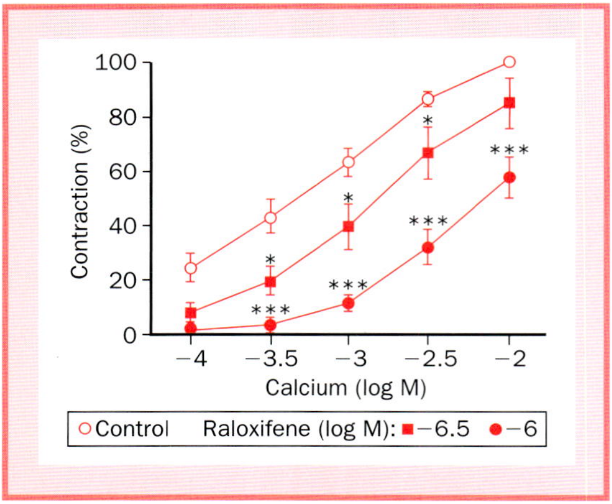

Figure 5.4
*The effect of raloxifene −6.5 (n = 7), −6 (n = 9) [log M] on the calcium concentration-dependent contraction curves in rabbit coronary arteries without endothelium compared with control (n = 11). Data are expressed as percentage of maximal contraction induced by calcium in controls (mean ± SEM). Significant differences in comparison with corresponding controls: *$p < 0.05$, ***$p < 0.001$. Redrawn from figure originally published in Figtree et al.*[34]

membrane when the extracellular potassium concentration is increased. Raloxifene relaxed coronary arterial rings contracted by high extracellular potassium both with and without endothelium. This suggests that it may have an inhibitory effect on potential-sensitive calcium channel activation in the smooth muscle cell. Raloxifene also induced relaxation of coronary arteries precontracted with $PGF_{2\alpha}$ (an agonist of receptor-operated calcium channels), indicating that raloxifene has relaxing effects on contraction induced by activation of both receptor-operated and potential-operated calcium channels. The shift of the calcium concentration-dependent contraction curve to the right by raloxifene suggests that raloxifene may be a calcium antagonist in these preparations, and may be a mechanism involved in the direct smooth muscle relaxation induced by raloxifene. Calcium antagonism may have been a result of decreased open probability of voltage-gated calcium channels secondary to a change in other ion conductances and consequent hyperpolarization. In order to investigate this, rings were incubated in the non-specific potassium channel blocker barium chloride. The shift of the calcium concentration-dependent contraction curve to the right was not reversed by incubation in barium chloride, suggesting that modulation of potassium channel conductance does not play a role in the direct calcium antagonistic effect of raloxifene.

Raloxifene took longer to induce relaxation than comparable studies using oestrogen.[6,39] Relaxation curves were performed over approximately 90 minutes versus 10–15 minutes for similar studies with oestrogen. The relaxant effect of raloxifene was not reversed over periods of up to 5 hours compared with oestrogen, for which initial precontraction levels were achieved after approximately 30 minutes. These observations are consistent with the finding of ER involvement in the endothelium-dependent relaxation by raloxifene. This is an effect that is not observed in vitro for oestrogen in this model[6] and is not involved in the calcium antagonistic effect. Further studies are needed to investigate this phenomenon because it may represent an advantage in long-term treatment. Steroid-induced events, which are mediated via classical intracellular receptors, occur over periods of minutes and hours. Thus, in our investigation, initial relaxation may be due to the early direct actions of raloxifene, followed by prolonged, ER-mediated relaxation.

In an identical way to the rabbit coronary work, similar results of a relaxing effect of raloxifene have been demonstrated in human coronary arteries.[40]

Conclusions

Coronary heart disease is one of the most important causes of morbidity and mortality in developed countries, in terms of both its prevalence and its human and economic cost. SERMs may have beneficial effects on the cardiovascular system in a similar way to oestrogen. Randomized studies in hormone therapy research are sadly lacking. This is largely the result of innumerable difficulties in conducting studies in a relatively elderly group of postmenopausal women. Choice of therapy is also a problem. It is hoped that with the development of SERMs, randomized studies on hard cardiovascular endpoints will be forthcoming. One such study is the RUTH study, which will report in 4–6 years. SERMs appear to have some favourable surrogate cardiovascular endpoints in both animals and humans, and it is now up to clinical scientists to prove, or otherwise, a cardiovascular benefit of long-term use of these agents in postmenopausal women. Further work in humans may identify a therapeutic role for raloxifene in reducing cardiovascular disease in postmenopausal women, and the significant mortality and morbidity associated with it.

References

1. Kuiper GG, Lemmen JG, Carlsson B et al. Interaction of estrogenic chemicals and phytoestrogens with estrogen receptor beta. *Endocrinology* 1998; **139**: 4252–63.
2. Jordan VC. Designer estrogens. *Sci Am* 1998; **279**: 60–7.
3. Stampfer MJ, Colditz GA, Willett WC et al. Postmenopausal estrogen therapy and cardiovascular disease. *N Engl J Med* 1991; **325**: 756–62.
4. Grodstein F, Stampfer MJ, Manson JE et al. Postmenopausal estrogen and progestin use and the risk of cardiovascular disease. *N Engl J Med* 1996; **335**: 453–61.
5. The Postmenopausal Estrogen/Progestin Interventions Trial Writing Group. Effects of estrogen or estrogen/progestin regimens on heart disease risk factors in postmenopausal women. *JAMA* 1995; **273**: 199–208.
6. Jiang C, Sarrel PM, Lindsay DC, Poole-Wilson PA, Collins P. Endothelium-independent relaxation of rabbit coronary artery by 17β-oestradiol in vitro. *Br J Pharmacol* 1991; **104**: 1033–7.
7. Sudhir K, Chou TM, Mullen WL et al. Mechanisms of estrogen-induced vasodilation: in vivo studies in canine coronary conductance and resistance arteries. *J Am Coll Cardiol* 1995; **26**(3): 807–14.
8. Chester AH, Jiang C, Borland JA, Yacoub MH, Collins P. Estrogen relaxes human epicardial coronary arteries through non-endothelium-dependent mechanisms. *Coron Artery Dis* 1995; **6**: 417–22.
9. Adams MR, Kaplan JR, Manuck SB et al. Inhibition of coronary artery atherosclerosis by 17-beta estradiol in ovariectomized monkeys. Lack of an effect of added progesterone. *Arteriosclerosis* 1990; **10**: 1051–7.
10. Jiang C, Poole-Wilson PA, Sarrel PM, Mochizuki S, Collins P, MacLeod KT. Effect of 17β-oestradiol on contraction, Ca^{2+} current and intracellular free Ca^{2+} in guinea-pig isolated cardiac myocytes. *Br J Pharmacol* 1992; **106**: 739–45.
11. Vedernikov YP, Liao QP, Jain V, Saade GR, Chwalisz K, Garfield RE. Effect of chronic treatment with 17beta-estradiol and progesterone on endothelium-dependent and endothelium-independent relaxation in isolated aortic rings from ovariectomized rats. *Am J Obstet Gynecol* 1997; **176**: 603–8.
12. Bell DR, Rensberger HJ, Koritnik DR, Koshy A. Estrogen pretreatment directly potentiates endothelium-dependent vasorelaxation of porcine coronary arteries. *Am J Physiol* 1995; **268**: H377–83.
13. Collins P, Shay J, Jiang C, Moss J. Nitric oxide accounts for dose-dependent estrogen-mediated coronary relaxation following acute estrogen withdrawal. *Circulation* 1994; **90**: 1964–8.
14. Gisclard V, Miller VM, Vanhoutte PM. Effect of 17β-estradiol on endothelium-dependent responses in the rabbit. *J Pharmacol Exp Ther* 1988; **244**: 19–22.
15. Williams SP, Shackelford DP, Iams SG, Mustafa SJ. Endothelium-dependent relaxation in estrogen-treated spontaneously hypertensive rats. *Eur J Pharmacol* 1988; **145**: 205–7.
16. Hayashi T, Fukuto JM, Ignarro LJ, Chaudhuri G. Basal release of nitric oxide from aortic rings is greater in female rabbits than in male rabbits: implications for atherosclerosis. *Proc Natl Acad Sci U S A* 1992; **89**: 11259–63.

17. Collins P, Rosano GMC, Sarrel PM et al. Estradiol-17β attenuates acetylcholine-induced coronary arterial constriction in women but not men with coronary heart disease. *Circulation* 1995; **92**: 24–30.

18. Wellman GC, Bonev AD, Nelson MT, Brayden JE. Gender differences in coronary artery diameter involve estrogen, nitric oxide, and Ca^{2+}-dependent K^{+} channels. *Circ Res* 1996; **79**: 1024–30.

19. Kim-Schulze S, McGowan KA, Hubchak SC et al. Expression of an estrogen receptor by human coronary artery and umbilical vein endothelial cells. *Circulation* 1996; **94**: 1402–7.

20. Shewmon DA, Stock JL, Abusamra LC, Kristan MA, Baker S, Heiniluoma KM. Tamoxifen decreases lipoprotein (a) in patients with breast cancer. *Metabolism* 1994; **43**: 531–2.

21. Grey AB, Stapleton JP, Evans MC, Reid IR. The effect of the anti-estrogen tamoxifen on cardiovascular risk factors in normal postmenopausal women. *J Clin Endocrinol Metab* 1995; **80**: 3191–5.

22. Love RR, Wiebe DA, Feyzi JM, Newcomb PA, Chappel RJ. Effects of tamoxifen on cardiovascular risk factors in postmenopasual women after 5 years of treatment. *J Natl Cancer Inst* 1994; **86**: 1534–9.

23. Walsh BW, Kuller LH, Wild RA et al. Effects of raloxifene on serum lipids and coagulation factors in healthy postmenopausal women. *JAMA* 1998; **279**: 1445–51.

24. Delmas PD, Bjarnason NH, Mitlak BH et al. Effects of raloxifene on bone mineral density, serum cholesterol concentrations, and uterine endometrium in postmenopausal women. *N Engl J Med* 1997; **337**: 1641–7.

25. Bass KM, Newschaffer CJ, Klag MJ, Bush TL. Plasma lipoprotein levels as predictors of cardiovascular death in women. *Arch Intern Med* 1993; **153**: 2209–16.

26. Miettinen M, Turpeinen O, Karvonen MJ, Elosuo R, Paavilainen E. Effect of cholesterol-lowering diet on mortality from coronary heart-disease and other causes. A twelve-year clinical trial in men and women. *Lancet* 1972; **ii**: 835–8.

27. Rutqvist LE, Mattsson A. Cardiac and thromboembolic morbidity among postmenopausal women with early-stage breast cancer in a randomized trial of adjuvant tamoxifen. Stockholm Breast Cancer Study Group. *J Natl Cancer Inst* 1993; **85**: 1398–406.

28. McDonald CC, Alexander FE, Whyte BW, Forrest AP, Stweart HJ. Cardiac and vascular morbidity in women receiving adjuvant tamoxifen for breast cancer in a randomised trial. The Scottish Cancer Trials Breast Group. *BMJ* 1995; **311**: 977–80.

29. Costantino J, Kuller L, Ives D et al. Coronary heart disease mortality and adjuvant tamoxifen therapy. *J Natl Cancer Inst* 1997; **89**(11): 747–9.

30. Cummings SR, Eckert S, Krueger KA et al. The effect of raloxifene on risk of breast cancer in postmenopausal women: results from the MORE randomized trial. Multiple Outcomes of Raloxifene Evaluation. *JAMA* 1999; **281**: 2189–97.

31. Barrett-Connor E, Wenger NK, Grady D et al. Coronary heart disease in women, randomized clinical trials, HERS and RUTH. *Maturitas* 1998; **31**: 1–7.

32. Clarkson TB, Anthony MS, Jerome CP. Lack of effect of raloxifene on coronary artery atherosclerosis of postmenopausal monkeys. *J Clin Endocrinol Metab* 1998; **83**(3): 721–6.

33. Bjarnason NH, Haarbo J, Byrjalsen I, Kauffman RF, Christiansen C. Raloxifene inhibits aortic accumulation of cholesterol in ovariectomized cholesterol-fed rabbits. *Circulation* 1997; **96**: 1964–9.

34. Rahimian R, Laher I, Dube G, Van-Breemen C. Estrogen and selective estrogen receptor modulator LY-117018 enhance release of nitric oxide in rat aorta. *J Pharmacol Exp Ther* 1997; **283**: 116–22 (Abstract).

35. Figtree GA, Lu Y-Q, Webb CM, Collins P. Raloxifene acutely relaxes rabbit coronary arteries in vitro by an estrogen receptor- and nitric oxide-dependent mechanism. *Circulation* 1999; **100**: 1095–101.

36. Palmer RMJ, Rees DD, Ashton DS, Moncada S. Larginine is the physiological precursor for the formation of nitric oxide in endothelium-dependent relaxation. *Biochem Biophys Res Commun* 1988; **153**: 1251–6.

37. Pohl U, Busse R. EDRF increases cyclic GMP in platelets during passage through the coronary vascular bed. *Circ Res* 1989; **65**: 1798–803.

38. Chen Z, Yuhanna IS, Galcheva-Gargova Z, Karas RH, Mendelsohn ME, Shaul PW. Estrogen receptor alpha mediates the nongenomic activation of endothelial nitric oxide synthase by estrogen. *J Clin Invest* 1999; **103**: 401–6.

39. Jiang C, Sarrel PM, Poole-Wilson PA, Collins P. Acute effect of 17β-estradiol on rabbit coronary artery contractile responses to endothelin-1. *Am J Physiol* 1992; **263**: H271–5.

40. Figtree GA, Lu-Y-Q, Webb CM, Collins P. Raloxifene acutely relaxes rabbit and human coronary arteries in vitro by an endothelium-dependent mechanism. *J Am Coll Cardiol* 1999; **33**(2) (Suppl A): 231 (Abstract).

6

Potential benefits of SERMs on the breast

Rita de Cassia M Dardes, V Craig Jordan

Oestrogen is an essential hormone for the development and maintenance of secondary female sex characteristics and control of the menstrual cycle. However, there is a link between its action and the development of some cancers. These cancers are called hormone-dependent, and are found most commonly in the breast. The development of selective oestrogen receptor modulators (SERMs), which can combat and prevent breast cancer, is the goal of current research. SERMs demonstrate potential benefits in the breast, skeleton and in coronary heart disease. In addition, the further development of agents to amplify the required actions of SERMs will enhance the benefits.

Discovery of the oestrogen receptor

In 1896, George Beatson demonstrated that oophorectomy in some women with breast cancer produced an improvement of the disease and prognosis.[1] However, the fact that only one-third of breast cancer patients showed benefit from the procedure[2] was explained, many years later, by the discovery of the oestrogen receptor (ER).

In 1923, Allen and Doisy[3] identified an 'estrus stimulating principle' in ovarian tissue that could be responsible for the development of breast cancer. Jensen and Jacobson subsequently demonstrated that $[^3H]E_2$ bound in oestrogen target tissues,[4] such as uterus, vagina and anterior pituitary, and proposed the concept of an ER to explain tissue-specific oestrogen action. Jensen, however, took the concept one step further by suggesting that the presence of ER in breast tumours could predict a response to endocrine ablation,[5] an hypothesis that was confirmed in large clinical studies worldwide.[6] Jensen's concept of the ER has been fundamental to the development of antioestrogens and the concept of selective ER modulation.[7–9]

This review will discuss the possible benefits of selective oestrogen receptor modulators (SERMs) on breast cancer and link basic research with clinical applications.

Early antioestrogens

Tamoxifen (***Figure 6.1***), an antioestrogen, was approved by the Food and Drug Administration for the treatment of advanced breast cancer in the USA in 1978. There are ten million woman years of clinical experience with tamoxifen and it is now the treatment of choice and the first drug to be used for reducing the incidence of breast cancer in high-risk women.[10–12] However, tamoxifen is not the first antioestrogen. Antioestrogens have been a pharmacological reality since 1958, but early compounds were toxic and there was little interest from the pharmaceutical industry for drug development. Lerner and co-workers[13] described the first non-steroidal antioestrogen, MER 25 (***Figure 6.1***), but it failed in clinical trials because large doses were required, causing serious side effects in the CNS.[14] The next compound, clomiphene or MRL-41 (***Figure 6.1***), a triphenylethylene, was found to be a postcoital contraceptive in rats,[15] but paradoxically was later developed as a fertility drug.[16] Nowadays, clomiphene is the standard therapy for treatment of infertility in anovulatory women. Tamoxifen or ICI 46,474 (***Figure 6.1***), a related triphenylethylene, was characterized as the pure *trans* isomer and was also found to be a postcoital contraceptive in rats but with potent antioestrogenic properties.[17–19] Although tamoxifen was tested for a number of clinical indications,[20] it is its successful application as a breast cancer therapy that has opened the door to new drug development.

Tamoxifen blocks the binding of oestradiol (competitive antagonist) to breast cancer ER[21] and prevents the growth of carcinogen-induced rat mammary tumours.[22,23] These observations promoted the development of

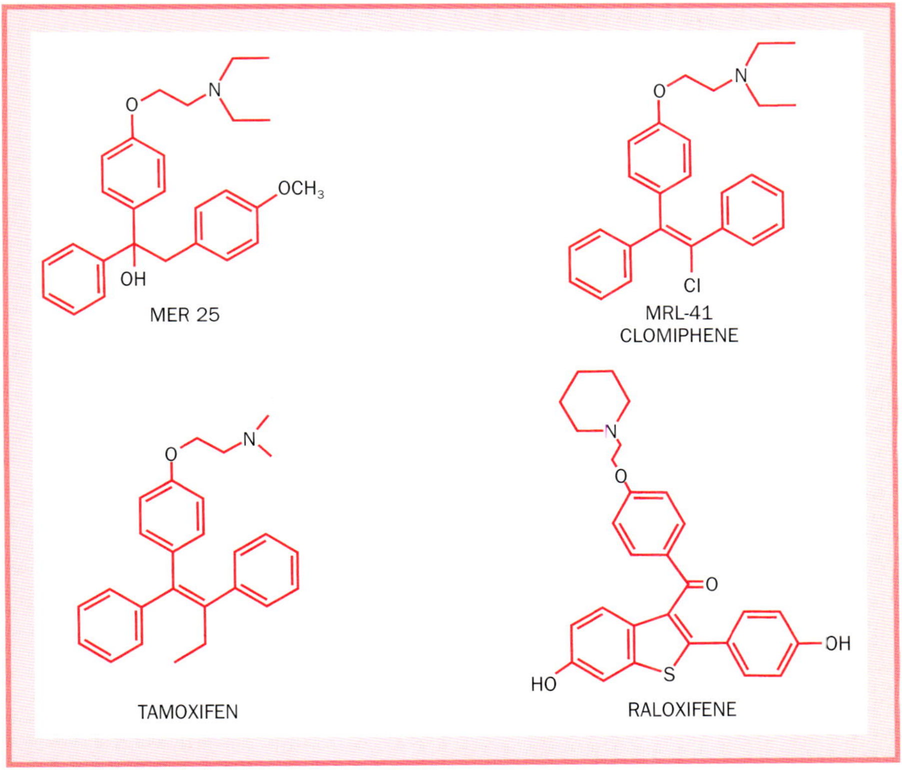

Figure 6.1
Structures of MER 25, clomiphene, tamoxifen and raloxifene. These non-steroidal antioestrogens are referred to in the text in more detail.

tamoxifen for breast cancer treatment and prevention. The clinical success of tamoxifen and the wealth of pharmacological knowledge provided by laboratory studies have changed our views about the applications of this group of drugs. Antioestrogens are now important tools to study the molecular pharmacology of hormone action. The goal is to understand the molecular mechanisms of selective ER modulation so that new drugs can be discovered.

Discovery of selective ER modulation

In the 1960s and 1970s, antioestrogenicity was correlated with antitumour activity. However, the finding that the compounds expressed oestrogenic properties, i.e. vaginal cornification and increased uterine weight in mice,[17,24] raised questions about the reasons for species specificity. One obvious possibility was species-specific metabolism, i.e. the mouse converts antioestrogens to oestrogens via novel metabolic pathways. However, no species-specific metabolic routes for known oestrogens[25,26] have been identified. Nevertheless, knowledge of the mouse model created a new dimension for study that ultimately led to the recognition of the target site actions of antioestrogens; a concept subsequently name selective ER modulation.

The ER-positive breast cancer cell line MCF-7[27] can be heterotransplanted into immune-deficient athymic mice, but the cells will only grow into tumours with oestrogen support. Paradoxically, tamoxifen, an oestrogen agonist in the mouse, does not support tumour growth[28] but stimulates mouse uterine growth with the same spectrum of tamoxifen metabolites present in both the mouse uterus and the human tumour.[29] To explain the selective actions of tamoxifen in different tissues of the same host, it was suggested that the ER complex could be interpreted as a stimulatory or inhibitory signal at different sites.[29] The concept was consolidated with experimental evidence from two further models. First, tamoxifen and raloxifene (***Figure 6.1***) maintain bone density in the ovariectomized rat, but both compounds inhibit oestradiol-stimulated uterine weight increase[30] and prevent carcinogen-induced mammary tumourigenesis.[31] Secondly, the finding that tamoxifen could partially stimulate the growth of a human endometrial carcinoma transplanted into athymic mice[32] provoked the investigation of two human tumours bi-transplanted in the same mouse to determine whether tamoxifen could inhibit oestrogen-stimulated growth of two tumours in the same host equally.[33] Tamoxifen demonstrated target site specificity; breast tumour growth was stopped but endometrial tumours continued to grow. Again, the range of tamoxifen metabolites was consistent in all target tissues despite the contrasting biological responses, so it was concluded that the ER complexes must be interpreted differently in different target tissues.

The mechanisms by which compounds exhibit tissue-specific oestrogenic and antioestrogenic effects are described in detail in Chapter 3.

Prevention of breast cancer with tamoxifen

The idea that breast cancer can be prevented by tamoxifen is based on animal

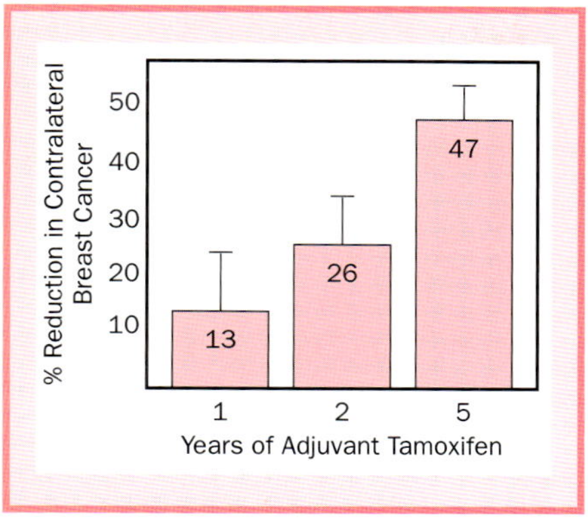

Figure 6.2
The relationship between the duration of adjuvant tamoxifen therapy in ER-positive premenopausal patients and the reduction in recurrence and death rate. A longer duration of treatment has a dramatic effect on patient survival. (Adapted from ref. 10.)

experiments,[22,34] which demonstrated that tamoxifen prevents mammary carcinogenesis. Additionally, there are 20 years of clinical experience showing that most women tolerate tamoxifen therapy because of the low occurrence of serious side effects.[35] Most importantly, the beneficial profile of oestrogen-like properties which maintain bone and decrease circulating LDL-cholesterol provides reassurance for women with respect to their risk of osteoporosis and coronary heart disease.

The link between endometrial carcinoma and tamoxifen is of major concern and has been studied intensively. There is some evidence that tamoxifen does not induce endometrial carcinoma, although its use is associated with a three- to fourfold increase in risk in postmenopausal women. Thus, the increase in the detection of endometrial cancer from one per thousand women per year to three per thousand women per year is consistent with the known rate of occult disease. In addition, the stage and grade of endometrial cancer observed in women taking tamoxifen is the same as that seen in the general population.[36,37] These findings provide support for the use of tamoxifen as a chemopreventive therapy for breast cancer.

Most importantly, the fact that tamoxifen (***Figure 6.2***) reduces the incidence of contralateral new breast cancers[38] makes it the primary agent to test in high-risk women. Tamoxifen is known to prevent new breast cancers in women with breast cancer but would women without breast cancer be willing to take the drug?

A major problem in the clinical identification of the 'high-risk woman' is the lack of knowledge of the interactions between various factors known to alter breast cancer risk since the majority of studies have focused on defining individual risk factors. Most women have a combination of factors which both increase and decrease risk, complicating the assessment of an individual's level of risk. Risk factors for breast cancer are illustrated in ***Table 6.1***.

We will describe three studies that have

Table 6.1
Magnitude of known breast cancer risk factors.

RR <2	RR 2–4	RR >4
Early menarche	Age >35 for first birth	Gene mutations
Late menopause	First-degree relative with breast cancer	Lobular carcinoma in situ
Nulliparity	Radiation exposure	Ductal carcinoma in situ
Proliferative benign disease	Prior breast cancer	
Obesity		
Alcohol use		
Hormone replacement		

RR, relative risk.

recently been published, which appear to provide conflicting information about the efficacy of tamoxifen as a preventive. However, it should be stressed that only the National Surgical Adjuvant Breast and Bowel Project (NSABP) study is a prospective randomized clinical trial with risk determined using a multiple risk factor evaluation profile.[39] These studies also reported results related to secondary endpoints, including the effects of tamoxifen on the incidence of fractures (osteoporosis) and cardiovascular protection, but we shall focus mainly on the effectiveness of tamoxifen as a preventive for breast cancer.

The Royal Marsden Pilot Study, which began in 1986,[40] was initially described as a pilot toxicology study which, subsequently, would become the vanguard for a nationwide clinical trial in Britain. In this preliminary study of 2494 women,[41] breast cancer prevention was not the primary endpoint and, as would be expected in an underpowered study, the results obtained did not demonstrate tamoxifen's efficacy as a preventive drug in women at high risk for breast cancer.

The Italian study, which began in 1992, was designed to determine whether tamoxifen was efficacious in preventing breast cancer. The original intent was to recruit 20 000 normal-risk women, but ultimately only 5408 hysterectomized women were studied because of concerns about an increased risk of endometrial carcinoma. These women, who were aged between 35 and 70 years, received

20 mg of tamoxifen per day for up to 5 years.[42] It should be noted that the participants were not at high risk of breast cancer; in addition, 1422 patients withdrew and only 149 women actually completed 5 years of treatment. The incidence of breast cancer did not differ between the groups (tamoxifen/placebo); however, it is very difficult to base conclusions on this very low number of participants.

The third study is the NSABP clinical trial,[11] which started in May 1992 in the USA and Canada. The stated goal of this study was to identify the potential benefits of tamoxifen as a breast cancer preventive. In 1997, this study analysed 13 388 high-risk participants between 35 and 75 years of age for breast cancer incidence. Endometrial biopsies were performed to evaluate the incidence of endometrial carcinoma. In addition, the effects of tamoxifen on cardiovascular disease and the incidence of osteoporotic fractures were observed.

The risk of invasive and non-invasive breast cancer was reduced in the tamoxifen group by 49% and 50%, respectively (***Figure 6.3***). When the ER status was analysed, a reduction of 69% per year was observed in the incidence of ER-positive tumours in the tamoxifen group while the effect of tamoxifen on the incidence of ER-negative tumours was similar to that of the placebo group (***Figure 6.4***). In terms of duration, 1 year of tamoxifen therapy resulted in a risk reduction of 33%, while 5 years' duration provided a 69% reduction in the risk of invasive breast cancer. These data demonstrate that 5 years of tamoxifen therapy is better than 1 year for the prevention of breast cancer.

Overall, the results of the NSABP trial, with its large study population, clearly demonstrate the benefit of tamoxifen for breast cancer prevention in high-risk women. These findings are consistent with laboratory observations[34] and with the contralateral breast cancer risk reduction seen with tamoxifen therapy.[10] Tamoxifen was approved in 1998 for the reduction of risk in pre- and postmenopausal women with a high risk of breast cancer.

Tamoxifen and raloxifene: from the laboratory to the clinic

Tamoxifen and raloxifene produce target site-specific effects in women. Both compounds produce antioestrogenic/antitumour actions on the incidence of breast cancer in well women.[43] Tamoxifen produces a 50% decrease in the incidence of breast cancer in both pre- and postmenopausal women at high risk.[11] The possibility that the oestrogen-like actions of SERMs on bone could justify the development of a drug for osteoporosis that would decrease the risk of breast cancer in postmenopausal women in general[7] has become a reality with the approval of raloxifene to prevent osteoporosis. An

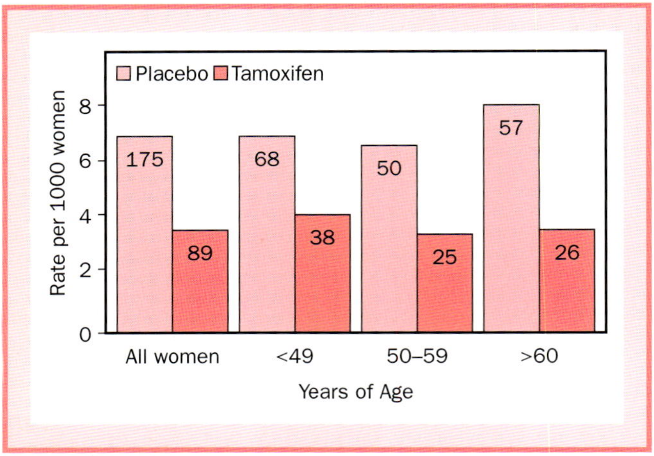

Figure 6.3
The overall reduction in invasive breast cancer observed in the NSABP tamoxifen prevention trial P-1; women at high risk for the disease were recruited to receive either tamoxifen (20 mg daily) or placebo. The women were also subdivided into age groups and the same reduction in the incidence of breast cancer was observed. The number of breast cancer occurrences is shown on the top of each histogram for each treatment arm. (Adapted from ref. 11.)

examination of all the clinical trial data in women treated with raloxifene to prevent osteoporosis demonstrates a 55% decrease in all breast cancers, but a decrease of 66% in invasive breast cancer.[44] In the MORE study,[45] ER-positive disease was reduced by 75%, comparable to the effects observed with tamoxifen,[11] but there was no effect on the incidence of ER-negative disease.

These data have prompted a direct comparison of the efficacy of raloxifene and tamoxifen for the prevention of breast cancer in a population of 22 000 high-risk postmenopausal women. In this trial, called the Study of Tamoxifen And Raloxifene (STAR), women will be randomized to receive either tamoxifen (20 mg daily) or raloxifene

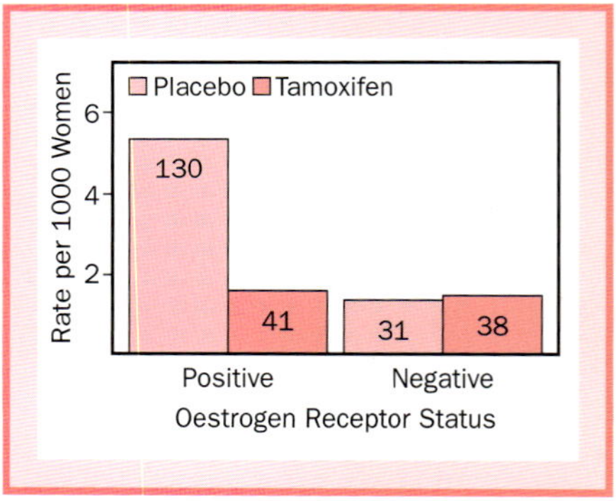

Figure 6.4
The incidence of ER-positive and ER-negative breast cancer in the placebo and tamoxifen-treated arms of the NSABP tamoxifen prevention trial P-1. The antioestrogen reduces the risk of developing ER-positive breast cancer but there is no change in the incidence of ER-negative breast cancer. The number of breast cancer occurrences is shown on the top of each histogram for each treatment arm. (Adapted from ref. 11.)

(60 mg daily) for 5 years with 2 years of follow-up after treatment stops.[43] Premenopausal women are not eligible because raloxifene has not been tested in premenopausal women.

Tamoxifen[46] and raloxifene[47] have beneficial effects on postmenopausal bone density and both drugs reduce the risk of fractures. Similarly, both tamoxifen[48] and raloxifene[49] have beneficial effects on low-density lipoprotein (LDL) cholesterol but do not lower high-density lipoprotein (HDL) cholesterol. Consistent with these effects, tamoxifen use has been associated with a decrease in fatal myocardial infarctions,[50] although these data have not been confirmed in women being treated for node negative breast cancer.[51] Nevertheless, raloxifene is to be tested in 10 000 women at risk for coronary heart disease in a trial called Raloxifene Use for The Heart (RUTH). Women will be randomized to placebo or raloxifene (60 mg) for 5 years.

Finally, it is important to state that tamoxifen is associated with a modest increase in endometrial cancer in postmenopausal women.[11,37] Although the initial publicity about endometrial cancer is now known to be overstated, this side effect is of concern to women. The STAR trial will compare and contrast the effects of tamoxifen and raloxifene on the endometrium and on the incidence of endometrial cancer. Routine endometrial biopsies will not be performed, but an evaluation will be made through self-reporting of symptoms and gynaecologic follow-up.[43] Specific subsets of women volunteers will be evaluated by transvaginal ultrasound and saline infusion for comparative endometrial thickness measurements. It is known that tamoxifen causes endometrial thickening by increasing stromal thickness[52,53] whereas this effect does not occur with raloxifene.[54] Results of the STAR trial will be available in 7 years' time.

The effective translation of selective oestrogen receptor modulation from the laboratory to the clinic has encouraged the search for the ideal targeted antioestrogen (***Figure 6.5***). The concept, first proposed in 1990,[7] has caused a paradigm shift in drug development so that multiple benefits can be obtained from a single intervention. Elucidation of the molecular mechanisms by which SERMs act will allow new targeted agents to be developed with a view to preventing the major diseases associated with advancing age after the menopause: osteoporosis, coronary heart disease, breast and endometrial cancer. It is even possible that such drugs could benefit or retard Alzheimer's disease if a brain-specific oestrogen is discovered. This will be the challenge for the twenty-first century.

Acknowledgements

We are extremely grateful to support from the

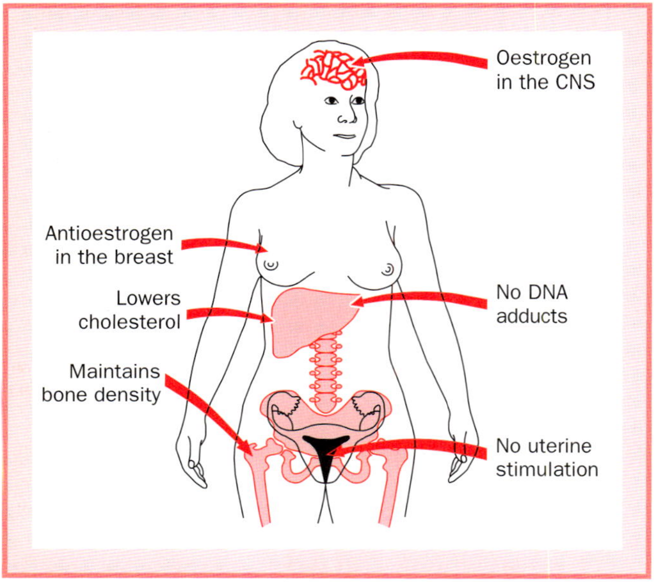

Figure 6.5
There is a need to develop the ideal targeted antioestrogen that could be used to prevent multiple diseases of the menopause. Tamoxifen and raloxifene both maintain bone density, lower cholesterol and are antioestrogens in the breast. There is no evidence that raloxifene produces DNA adducts in experimental systems and the STAR trial will establish the extent of uterine stimulation versus tamoxifen. The challenge is to develop a compound that is also an oestrogen in the CNS.

Lynn Sage Breast Cancer Research Foundation of Northwestern Memorial Hospital and CAPES – research programme from the Ministry of Education-Brasilia, DF, Brazil.

References

1. Beatson GT. On the treatment of inoperable cases of carcinoma of the mamma: suggestions for a new method of treatment with illustrative cases. *Lancet* 1896; **ii**: 104–7.
2. Boyd S. On oophorectomy in cancer of the breast. *Br Med J* 1900; **ii**: 1161–7.
3. Allen E, Doisy EA. An ovarian hormone: preliminary report on its localization, extraction and partial purification and action in test animals. *JAMA* 1923; **81**: 819–21.
4. Jensen EV, Jacobson HI. Basic guides to the mechanism of estrogen action. *Recent Prog Horm Res* 1962; **18**: 387–414.
5. Jensen EV, Block GE, Smith S, Kyser K, DeSombre ER. Estrogen receptors and breast cancer response to adenalectomy. *Natl Cancer Inst Monogr* 1971; **34**: 55–70.
6. McGuire WL, Carbone PP, Volmer EP. *Estrogen Receptors in Human Breast Cancer.* Raven Press: New York, 1975.
7. Lerner LJ, Jordan VC. Development of antiestrogens and their use in breast cancer: eighth BF Cain Memorial Award. *Cancer Res* 1990; **50**: 4177–89.

8. Jordan VC (ed). *Long-term Tamoxifen Treatment for Breast Cancer.* University of Wisconsin Press: Madison, WI, 1994.

9. Jordan VC. Designer estrogens. *Sci Am* 1998; **279**: 60–7.

10. Early Breast Cancer Trialists' Collaborative Group. Tamoxifen for early breast cancer: an overview of the randomized trials. *Lancet* 1998; **351**: 1451–67.

11. Fisher B, Costantino JP, Wickerham DL et al. Tamoxifen for prevention of breast cancer: report of the National Surgical Adjuvant Breast and Bowel Project P-1 Study. *J Natl Cancer Inst* 1998; **90**: 1371–88.

12. Osborne CK. Tamoxifen in the treatment of breast cancer. *N Engl J Med* 1998; **339**: 1609–18.

13. Lerner LJ, Holthaus JF, Thompson CR. A nonsteroidal estrogen antagonist 1-(p-2-diethylaminoethoxyphenyl)-1-phenyl-2-p-methoxyphenyl-ethanol. *Endocrinology* 1958; **63**: 295–318.

14. Lerner LJ. The first non-steroidal antioestrogen – MER 25. In: Sutherland RL, Jordan VC (eds). *Non Steroidal Antioestrogens: Molecular Pharmacology and Antitumour Activity.* Academic Press: Sydney, 1981: 1–6.

15. Holtkamp DE, Greslin SC, Root CA, Lerner LJ. Gonadotropin inhibiting and antifecundity effects of chloramiphene. *Proc Soc Exp Biol Med* 1960; **105**: 197–201.

16. Huppert LC. Induction of ovulation with clomiphene citrate. *Fertil Steril* 1979; **31**: 1–8.

17. Harper MJK, Walpole AL. A new derivative of triphenylethylene: effect on implantation and mode of action in rats. *J Reprod Fertil* 1967; **13**: 101–19.

18. Harper MJK, Walpole AL. Mode of action of ICI 46,474 in preventing implantation in rats. *J Endocrinol* 1967; **37**: 83–92.

19. Labsetwar AP. Role of estrogen in ovulation. A study using the estrogen antagonist ICI46, 474. *Endocrinology* 1970; **87**: 542–51.

20. Jordan VC. The development of tamoxifen for breast cancer therapy: a tribute to the late Arthur L. Walpole (invited feature). *Breast Cancer Res Treat* 1988; **11**: 197–209.

21. Jordan VC, Koerner S. Tamoxifen (ICI46, 474) and the human carcinoma 8S oestrogen receptor. *Eur J Cancer* 1975; **11**: 205–6.

22. Jordan VC. Antitumor activity of the antioestrogen ICI46, 474 (tamoxifen) in the dimethylbenzanthracene (DMBA)-induced rat mammary carcinoma model. *J Steroid Biochem* 1974; **5**: 354.

23. Jordan VC. Effect of tamoxifen (ICI 46, 474) on initiation and growth of DMBA-induced rat mammary carcinomas. *Eur J Cancer* 1976; **12**: 419–24.

24. Terenius L. Structure–activity relationships of antioestrogens with regard to interaction with 17 β oestradiol in the mouse uterus and vagina. *Acta Endocrinol* 1971; **66** (suppl): 431–47.

25. Lyman SD, Jordan VC. Metabolism of nonsteroidal antiestrogens. In: Jordan VC (ed). *Estrogen/antiestrogen Action and Breast Cancer Therapy.* University of Wisconsin Press: Madison, WI, 1986: 191–219.

26. Robinson SP, Langan-Fahey SM, Jordan VC. Implications of tamoxifen metabolism in the athymic mouse for the study of antitumour effects upon human breast cancer xenografts. *Eur J Cancer Clin Oncol* 1989; **25**: 1769–76.

27. Levenson AS, Jordan VC. MCF-7: The first hormone responsive breast cancer cell line (Perspectives in Cancer Research). *Cancer Res* 1997; **57**: 3071–8.

28. Osborne CK, Hobbs K, Clark GM. Effects of estrogens and antiestrogens on growth of

human breast cancer cells in athymic nude mice. *Cancer Res* 1985; **45**: 584–90.

29. Jordan VC, Robinson SP. Species specific pharmacology of antiestrogens: role of metabolism. *Fed Proc* 1987; **46**: 1870–4.

30. Jordan VC, Phelps E, Lindgren JU. Effects of antiestrogens on bone in castrated and intact female rats. *Breast Cancer Res Treat* 1987; **10**: 31–5.

31. Gottardis MM, Jordan VC. The antitumor actions of keoxifene (raloxifene) and tamoxifen in the *N*-nitrosomethylurea-induced rat mammary carcinoma model. *Cancer Res* 1987; **47**: 4020–4.

32. Satyaswaroop PG, Zaino RJ, Mortel R. Estrogen-like effects of tamoxifen on endometrial carcinoma transplanted in nude mice. *Cancer res* 1984; **44**: 4006–10.

33. Gottardis MM, Robinson SP, Satyaswaroop PG, Jordan VC. Contrasting actions of tamoxifen on endometrial and breast tumor growth in the athymic mouse. *Cancer Res* 1988; **48**: 812–15.

34. Jordan VC, Jaspan T. Tamoxifen as an antitumour agent: oestrogen binding as a predictive test for tumour response. *J Endocrinol* 1976; **68**: 453–60.

35. Furr BJA, Jordan VC. The pharmacology and clinical uses of tamoxifen. *Pharmacol Ther* 1984; **25**: 127–205.

36. Assikis VJ, Neven P, Jordan VC, Vergote I. A realistic clinical perspective of tamoxifen and endometrial carcinogenesis. *Eur J Cancer* 1996; **32**: 1464–76.

37. Fisher B, Costantino JP, Redmond CK, Fisher ER, Wickerham DL, Cronin WM. Endometrial cancer in tamoxifen treated breast cancer patients. Findings from the National Surgical Adjuvant Breast and Bowel Project (NSABP) *J Cancer Inst* 1994; **86**: 527–37.

38. Cuzick J, Baum M. Tamoxifen and contralateral breast cancer. *Lancet* 1985; 282.

39. Gail MH, Brinton LA, Byar DP et al. Projecting individualized probabilities of developing breast cancer for white females who are being examined annually. *J Natl Cancer Inst* 1989; **81**: 1879–86.

40. Powles TJ, Hickish T, Kanis JA, Tidy VA, Ashley S. Effect of tamoxifen on bone mineral density measured by dual energy x-ray absorptiometry in healthy premenopausal and postmenopausal women. *J Clin Oncol* 1996; **14**: 78–84.

41. Powles TJ, Eeles R, Ashley SE et al. Interim analysis of the incident breast cancer in the Royal Marsden Hospital tamoxifen randomized chemoprevention trial. *Lancet* 1998; **362**: 98–101.

42. Veronesi U, Maisonneuve P, Costa A et al. Prevention of breast cancer with tamoxifen: preliminary findings from the Italian randomized trial among hysterectomized women. *Lancet* 1998; **362**: 93–7.

43. Jordan VC, Morrow M. Tamoxifen, raloxifene and the prevention of breast cancer. *Endocrine Rev* 1999; **20**(3): 253–78.

44. Jordan VC, Glusman JE, Eckert S et al. Raloxifene reduces incident primary breast cancers. Integrated data from multicenter double blind, placebo controlled randomized trials in postmenopausal women. *Breast Cancer Res Treat* 1998; **50**: 227 (Abstract 2).

45. Cummings SR, Eckert S, Krueger KA et al. The effect of raloxifene on risk of breast cancer in postmenopausal women: results from MORE randomized trial. Multiple Outcomes of Raloxifene Evaluation. *JAMA* 1999; **281**: 2189–97.

46. Love RR, Mazess RB, Barden HS et al. Effects of tamoxifen on bone mineral density in postmenopausal women with breast cancer. *N Engl J Med* 1992; **326**: 885–6.

47. Delmas PD, Bjarnason NH, Mitlak BH et al. Effects of raloxifene on bone mineral density, serum cholesterol concentrations and uterine endometrium in postmenopausal women. *N Engl J Med* 1997; **337**: 1641–7.

48. Love RR, Wiebe DA, Newcomb PA et al. Effects of tamoxifen on cardiovascular risk factors in postmenopausal women. *Ann Intern Med* 1991; **115**: 860–4.

49. Walsh BW, Kuller LH, Wild RA et al. Effects of raloxifene on serum lipids and coagulation factors in healthy postmenopausal women. *JAMA* 1998; **279**: 1445–51.

50. McDonald CC, Alexander FE, Whyte BW, Forest AP, Steward HJ. Cardiac and vascular morbidity in women receiving adjuvant tamoxifen for breast cancer in a randomized trial. *Br Med J* 1995; **311**: 977–80.

51. Costantino JP, Kuller LH, Ives DG, Fisher B, Dignam J. Coronary heart disease mortality and adjuvant tamoxifen therapy. *J Natl Cancer Inst* 1997; **89**: 776–82.

52. Goldstein SR. Unusual ultrasonographic appearance of the uterus in patients receiving tamoxifen. *Am J Obstet Gynecol* 1994; **49**: 447–51.

53. Decensi A, Fontana V, Bruno S, Costa A. Effect of tamoxifen on endometrial proliferation. *J Clin Oncol* 1996; **14**: 434–40.

54. Boss SM, Huster WJ, Neild JA, Glant MD, Eisenhut CC, Draper MW. Effect of raloxifene hydrochloride on the endometrium of postmenopausal women. *Am J Obstet Gynecol* 1997; **177**: 1458–64.

7

Effects of SERMs on symptoms of the menopause

Martina Dören

Selective oestrogen receptor modulators such as raloxifene may slightly increase vasomotor symptoms of the menopause (e.g. hot flushes). Limited evidence suggests that raloxifene does not interfere with cognitive function or health-related quality of life aspects such as mood, general well-being, sexuality and urogenital ageing.

Introduction

Contemporary psychometric instruments designed to reflect the complexity of symptoms that menopausal women may experience have extended beyond the Kupperman menopausal index, emphasizing the presence of vasomotor symptoms.[1] Various comprehensive, validated and reliable instruments based on self-reported evaluations have been developed which reflect a range of emotional and physical symptoms of menopausal women and allow for factor analysis.[2–4] Many physical, emotional and social aspects determine the quality of life of postmenopausal women, a term addressing not only specific health-related issues of this period of life but reflective of an individual's overall satisfaction with life and general sense of well-being.[5,6]

Vasomotor symptoms

According to surveys, hot flushes (or flashes) are the most common self-reported symptom of peri- and postmenopausal women of European descent experiencing natural menopause or menopause due to medical interventions including oophorectomy or chemotherapy, where up to 85% of menopausal women experience flushes.[7–13] Substantially lower prevalences have been reported for Asian women,[14,15] and hot flushes may not be perceived at all in some populations.[16] However, whether questionnaires designed for European and North American women are applicable to and reflective of the symptomatology of non-European populations is debatable. Flushes are most prevalent in the first two postmenopausal years, becoming less frequent over time, but may persist in the very elderly. They may be experienced in premenopausal women, in pregnancy and in the postpartum period as well as in men with abrupt loss of testicular function. Flushes may occur in conjunction with various malignant diseases, neurological disorders, anxiety, emotional flushing (blushing), chronic stress, alcohol, and many drugs and food additives.[17]

Transient thermoregulatory and cardiovascular changes that accompany hot flushes are well documented,[18–20] as are alterations in respiration.[21] Hot flushes may be described as sudden, transient sensations ranging from warmth to heat, starting at the chest and face, spreading over the body, and finally followed by perspiration. Many other physical and emotional phenomena may be associated with flushes. Thus, the sequence of events that characterizes a hot flush seems to be the result of a temporary activity change in thermoregulation controlled by the hypothalamus, with a sudden drop in set-point temperature involving consecutive mechanisms of heat loss and, finally, heat conservation. The physiological basis for the wide range of inter- and intra-individual flush patterns has yet to be definitively explained. Essentially it is unknown what causes the transient temperature adjustments. It has been suggested that a sudden decrease in the endogenous concentrations of oestradiol and oestrone may trigger hot flushes, though probably not the presence of low levels of either sex steroid per se. Episodic luteinizing hormone (LH) and gonadotropin-releasing hormone (GnRH) release are not necessary for hot flushes to occur. However, a temporal correlation does exist between LH measured in the peripheral circulation and the onset of flushes. The serum concentration of various ovarian, adrenal, pituitary, and hypothalamic steroids and peptides may change in association with flushes. The hypotheses discussed predominantly to explain flushes include α-adrenergic mechanisms, β-endorphin and GnRH release, all of which may be modulated by reproductive hormones.[20,22,23]

Successful management of hot flushes in some women can be achieved by modifications of behaviour and/or environmental factors such as changes of clothing, room temperature, or avoidance of beverages containing alcohol or caffeine. Paced respiration and muscle relaxation,[24] acupuncture[25] and physical exercise[26] have all been reported to be helpful in the non-hormonal management of flushes.

Symptomatic relief may be achieved in the majority of women with oestrogen replacement therapy (ERT), which is the most effective medical treatment. Essentially, all types of oestrogens, including ethinyloestradiol, administered via the oral or parenteral route are effective in alleviating or eliminating hot flushes in a dose-dependent fashion. For example, in a double-blind, placebo-controlled crossover trial lasting 3 months, flushes were reduced by 90% in women taking 1.25 mg conjugated equine oestrogens daily compared with 62% in the placebo group.[27] Thus, placebo is also effective as demonstrated by other trials. There seems to be no difference if a sequential progestin such as medroxyprogesterone acetate is added to oestrogen replacement with conjugated equine oestrogens.[28] However, oral hormone replacement therapy (HRT) consisting of continuously combined 1 mg oestradiol and 0.5 mg norethisterone acetate may be superior to the same dose of unopposed oestradiol and placebo.[29] Megestrol acetate and medroxyprogesterone acetate have been shown to reduce hot flushes.[30]

A variety of other substances may also alleviate hot flushes: clonidine, lofexidine and α-methyl-dopa, probably due to α-adrenergic properties;[31–33] bellergal, which is a combination of belladonna alkaloids; ergotamine tartrate; phenobarbital;[34] and veraliprid, a dopamine antagonist.[35] There is inconclusive evidence as to whether propranolol, a peripherally and centrally acting beta-receptor blocker, is beneficial due to conflicting results from placebo-controlled, randomized, double-blind trials.[36,37] Phytoestrogens provide another approach to reduce hot flushes. Isolated soy protein with a standardized content of isoflavones has been shown to reduce flushes and was superior to casein placebo in a randomized, double-blind, 3-month trial of natural and surgically postmenopausal symptomatic women.[38] However, one double-blind, randomized, crossover trial for 2 × 12 weeks in postmenopausal women reported the greatest flush reduction in women on wheat rather than soy or linseed diets.[39] Ingredients of black cohosh (*Cimicifuga racemosa*) may also reduce flushes in pre- and postmenopausal women.[40,41]

Hot flushes are a well-known side-effect of various medications. They frequently occur in pre- and postmenopausal breast cancer patients treated with tamoxifen, a triphenylethylene tissue-specific antioestrogen. In a long-term double-blind, randomized, placebo-controlled trial involving 13 388 pre- and postmenopausal women above the age of 35 years at increased risk of breast cancer, 20 mg tamoxifen daily was reported to be associated with hot flushes in 45.7% of pre- and postmenopausal women compared with 28.7% in the placebo group within the average follow-up of almost 6 years.[42]

Raloxifene, a benzothiophene analogue which acts as a selective oestrogen receptor modulator (SERM), was reported to increase the incidence of hot flushes in postmenopausal women including those who had only mild climacteric symptoms prior to the trial.[43,44] There appears to be a dose–response relationship since the daily dose of 120 mg was associated with a higher incidence of hot flushes compared with the 60 mg dose.[45] Another double-blind, randomized, placebo-controlled 2-year trial of postmenopausal women with absent or only mild climacteric symptoms prior to enrolment reported an increase of flushes both for the group receiving 60 mg raloxifene daily and the placebo group, 26.3% versus 22.7%; this difference was not statistically significant.[45] There was no evidence that women assigned to this dose of raloxifene were more likely to discontinue the study because of flushes compared with placebo. However, pooled data show that the overall incidence of flushes was significantly higher in women treated with raloxifene 60 mg compared to either sequential or continuous combined HRT consisting of CEE 0.625 mg daily and a progestogen (medroxyprogesterone acetate or norgestrel), unopposed CEE 0.625 mg, or placebo.[46] The self-reported severity of flushes including the initial treatment phase was mild to moderate in 22.5% and severe in 2.1% of women assigned to raloxifene 60 mg. Figures for placebo were 16.4% and 1.9% respectively. The difference between raloxifene and placebo was significant only for the initial six months. Thereafter, the incidence of flushes was 7.6% for raloxifene 60 mg and 6.9% for placebo. The proportion of women who discontinued the placebo-controlled trials due to flushes was similar in women assigned to placebo or raloxifene. There was no difference in daytime and nightime sweats whether raloxifene, placebo or HRT was used for treatment, although the difference when CEE was used was almost significant. The frequency of insomnia was not different across all groups.[46] The large MORE trial, a prospective long-term secondary prevention trial in late postmenopausal women with osteoporosis, confirmed that use of raloxifene is associated with an increased rate of hot flushes – 9.7% (60 mg dose) and 11.6% (120 mg dose) compared with placebo (6.4%).[47] In this study, 0.6% and 0.1% of the discontinuations were due to flushes in the pooled raloxifene groups and the placebo group respectively. It was beyond the scope of an exploratory trial of raloxifene use in premenopausal women to address the issue of hot flushes.[48] In a hot flush rat model, raloxifene as well as tamoxifen demonstrated mixed oestrogen agonist/ antagonist activities.[49] Preliminary data suggest that idoxifene, another SERM, is also associated with increased flushes as demonstrated in osteopenic women below the age of 65 years in a double-blind, randomized, placebo-controlled 3-month trial.[50] It is unknown why women taking SERMs experience hot flushes, but it is thought that the antioestrogenic properties of these compounds are responsible for this effect.

Further quality of life aspects

Cognitive function

There are plausible biological mechanisms by which oestrogens might improve cognition; most of the evidence is based on preclinical (animal) research.[51] Conflicting results of observational studies and clinical trials have recently been systematically analysed to elucidate the effects of ERT on cognition in postmenopausal and surgically menopausal women.[52,53] The authors concluded that ERT does not improve cognitive function and its use should not be recommended for prevention of Alzheimer's disease. An improvement in climacteric symptoms such as hot flushes may be responsible for the inconsistently demonstrated improvement of cognitive tests after administration of exogenous oestrogens. However, there is other evidence to suggest that vasomotor symptoms and cognitive performance are unrelated, as examined in hysterectomized postmenopausal women without use of HRT.[54] Recently, further results of the Postmenopausal Estrogen/Progestin Interventions (PEPI) trial regarding aspects of cognitive function were reported.[55] A questionnaire aimed at addressing forgetfulness, differences in concentration, and distraction did not demonstrate significant differences in this cohort of non-demented, healthy middle-aged women randomized to either unopposed conjugated equine oestrogen (CEE), CEE plus a sequential progestin (medroxyprogesterone acetate (MPA) or micronized progesterone), continuous combined CEE and MPA, or placebo. However, there was a trend towards less forgetfulness in women assigned to any combined oestrogen and progestin therapy compared with unopposed oestrogen replacement. Additionally, there was some indication that women assigned to CEE and sequential MPA were less likely to report symptoms indicative of concentration problems compared with the continuous combined group.[55] As various methodological limitations apply to most of the published observational studies and clinical trials it seems premature to state that ERT/HRT (hormone replacement therapy) is effective in improving the cognitive performance of postmenopausal women.

It was recently shown that raloxifene did not adversely affect cognitive function or mood in postmenopausal women treated daily with 60 or 120 mg of this compound in a double-blind, randomized, placebo-controlled 1-year trial involving 143 non-demented patients between the ages of 55 and 76 years with an established diagnosis of osteoporosis.[56] Validated instruments such as the memory assessment clinics cognitive test battery, which measures independent parameters of learning and memory, the Walter Reed performance assessment battery, which examines aspects of attention, information-processing speed and efficiency, and reaction time, and the Geriatric Depression Scale were applied in this clinical trial.

Animal experiments to elucidate the impact of raloxifene on the central nervous system have yielded findings suggestive of both oestrogenic and antioestrogenic properties. Raloxifene was shown to have similar effects to oestradiol on the outgrowth of neurites in rat PC12 cells in vitro, pre-primed with nerve growth factor in order to induce expression of both ERα and ERβ. In this study, raloxifene did not block the neurite growth of simultaneously oestradiol-treated PC12 cells; the combined effect of oestradiol- and raloxifene-induced neurite outgrowth was greater than the effect of either substance alone.[57] In ovariectomized rats, benzothiophene SERMs similar to raloxifene induced identical patterns of hippocampal mRNA expression, suggestive of oestrogen agonistic properties. However, there is some experimental evidence to suggest anti-oestrogenic effects of raloxifene in the rat brain. Raloxifene may retard oestrogen-induced peroxidase accumulation in the brain with ageing[58] and it may antagonize oestrogen-induced changes of luteinizing hormone[59] and oestrogen-stimulated expression of hypothalamic progesterone receptor mRNA.[60] Whether any of these findings are of clinical relevance for postmenopausal women is unknown.

Well-being and mood

Psychological well-being in the postmenopause is not consistently different from that of premenopausal women, as demonstrated in large random samples of perimenopausal women,[61–63] and the menopause is not necessarily associated with an increased risk of depressive mood. Rather, social and family factors have been found to be more important in the aetiology of depressive symptomatology.[9,62] Most investigations, except for a few clinical trials[55,64] which assessed the effects of HRT on mood, did not control for vasomotor symptoms as a confounding factor, including a recent meta-analysis;[65] this may be relevant in view of the inverse correlation between vasomotor symptoms and both general well-being[66,67] and mood.[68] Mood is also known to interfere with performance on cognitive assessment batteries.[69] Very little is known about the impact of SERMs on mood. There seemed to be no difference in depression and instability of mood in women treated with raloxifene or placebo in a pooled analysis of double-blind, randomized trials.[47] There was also no alteration in the state of mood of postmenopausal women with osteoporosis using raloxifene,[56] as assessed by validated instruments, and no significant difference in self-reported quality of life, including depression in women at increased risk for breast cancer using tamoxifen or placebo.[42]

Sexuality

Similar limitations and considerations to those discussed previously apply for the issue of sexuality and menopause[70] and the possible potential for ERT/HRT in postmenopausal women with perceived impaired quality of sexual life. However, in surgically menopausal women, suddenly deprived of both endogenous ovarian oestrogen and androgen production, the benefits of HRT including (methyl)testosterone preparations, have been demonstrated.[71] Published preliminary findings suggest that sexual life seems not to be impaired in women at increased risk for breast cancer who are taking tamoxifen.[42]

Urogenital symptoms

Vulvovaginal itching, burning and dyspareunia are commonly related to postmenopausal oestrogen deficiency in the context of atrophic changes of the epithelium, connective tissue, blood supply and muscular tissue support. They are often associated with urinary frequency, dysuria and incontinence. A variety of medical problems such as diabetes[72] and other, not necessarily medical, problems may also be of importance to explain these symptoms, which some women find difficult to communicate.[73] Oestrogen replacement therapy subjectively improves urinary incontinence; however, clinical investigations using objective measurements including urodynamic assessments of incontinence mostly failed to support a role for ERT.[74] There are inconsistent data from the few prospective, controlled clinical trials and epidemiological studies addressing the relationship between HRT and various types of incontinence, the prevalence of which seems to vary widely across age groups and populations.[75–77] Other symptoms of both urinary and vaginal atrophy, excluding incontinence, frequently respond to local and systemic therapy with various types of oestrogens over a wide dose range.[78]

Emerging pooled data on the impact of raloxifene on symptoms of the so-called complex of urogenital ageing suggest that this compound does not differ compared with placebo in its effect on vaginal dryness, dyspareunia and decreased libido.[47] Use of tamoxifen seems to be associated with an increase in vaginal discharge,[42] the clinical relevance of which is unknown.

In conclusion, given the multitude of medical conditions associated with the phenomenon of a hot flush and its yet not completely defined pathophysiology, it is uncertain whether flushes, as a main symptom of the climacteric period in women of European descent, are exclusively due to the decline of ovarian function. A variety of different pharmacological agents may cause and alleviate flushes. The most widely used medical treatment is HRT. SERMs may cause or increase already perceived flushes in less than 10% of women. It is premature to conclude that oestrogen (hormone) replacement therapy is proven to be beneficial for cognitive function. Preliminary data suggest that cognitive function and mood may not be altered by SERMs. Aspects of general well-being including mood, sexuality and symptoms of urogenital ageing also deserve further attention in the context of controlled clinical trials to elucidate the potential of both medical treatments.

References

1. Kupperman HS, Wetchler BB, Blatt MH. Contemporary therapy of the menopausal syndrome. *JAMA* 1959; **171**: 1627–37.
2. Hunter M, Battersby R, Whitehead M. Relationship between psychological symptoms, somatic complaints and menopausal status. *Maturitas* 1986; **8**: 217–28.
3. Hilditch JR, Lewis J, Peter A et al. A menopause-specific quality of life questionnaire: development and psychometric properties. *Maturitas* 1996; **24**: 161–75.
4. Greene JG. Constructing a standard climacteric scale. *Maturitas* 1998; **29**: 25–31.
5. Shumaker SA, Anderson RT, Czajkowski SM. Psychological tests and scales. In: Spilker B (ed). *Quality of Life Assessments in Clinical Trials.* Raven Press: New York, 1990: 95–113.
6. Wiklund I. Methods of assessing the impact of climacteric complaints on quality of life. *Maturitas* 1998; **29**: 41–50.
7. Hammar M, Berg G, Fåhraeus L, Larsson-Cohn U. Climacteric symptoms in an unselected sample of Swedish women. *Maturitas* 1984; **6**: 345–50.
8. Kaufert P. Women and their health in the middle years: a Manitoba project. *Soc Sci Med* 1984; **3**: 1029–30.
9. Ballinger SE. Psychosocial stress and symptoms of menopause: a comparative study of menopause clinic patients and non-patients. *Maturitas* 1985; 7: 315–27.
10. McKinlay JB, McKinlay SM, Brambilla D. The relative contribution of endocrine changes and social circumstances in mid-aged women. *J Health Soc Behav* 1987; **28**: 345–63.
11. Holte A. Prevalence of climacteric complaints

in a representative sample of middle-aged women in Oslo, Norway. *J Psychosom Obstet Gynecol* 1991; **12**: 303–17.

12. Hunter M. The South-East England longitudinal study of the climacteric and postmenopause. *Maturitas* 1992; **14**: 117–26.

13. Oldenhave A, Jaszmann LJB, Haspels AA, Everaerd WTAM. Impact of climacteric on well-being: a survey based on 5.213 women aged 39 to 60 years old. *Am J Obstet Gynecol* 1993; **168**: 772–80.

14. Lock M, Kaufert P, Gilbert P. Cultural construction of the menopausal syndrome: the Japanese case. *Maturitas* 1988; **10**: 317–32.

15. Boulet MJ, Oddens BJ, Lehert P et al. Climacteric and menopause in seven south-east Asian countries. *Maturitas* 1994; **19**: 157–76.

16. Beyene Y. *From Menarche to Menopause: Reproductive Lives of Peasant Women in Two Cultures.* State University of New York Press: Albany, 1989.

17. Mohyi D, Tabassi K, Simon J. Differential diagnosis of hot flashes. *Maturitas* 1997; **27**: 203–14.

18. Molnar GW. Body temperatures during menopausal hot flashes. *J Appl Physiol* 1975; **38**: 499-503.

19. Tataryn IV, Meldrum DR, Lu KH et al. LH, FSH, and skin temperature during menopausal hot flush. *J Clin Endocrinol Metab* 1979; **49**: 823–5.

20. Kronenberg F. Hot flashes. In: Lobo RA (ed). *Treatment of Postmenopausal Women: Basic and Clinical Aspects.* Raven Press: New York, 1994: 97–117.

21. Woodward S, Greville HW, Freedman RR. Ventilatory response during menopausal hot flashes. *Menopause* 1995; **2**: 81–8.

22. Casper RF, Yen SSC. Neuroendocrinology of menopausal flushes: an hypothesis of fluid mechanism. *Clin Endocrinol* 1985; **22**: 293–312.

23. Genazzani AR, Stomati M, Spinetti A et al. Neuroendocrinology of the climacteric period and hormonal replacement therapy. In: Wren BG (ed). *Progress in the Management of the Menopause.* Parthenon Publishing: Lancaster, 1997: 380–4.

24. Germaine L, Freedman RR. Behavioral treatment of menopausal hot flushes: evaluation by objective methods. *J Consult Clin Psychol* 1984; **52**: 1072–9.

25. Wyon Y, Lindgren R, Lundeberg T, Hammar M. Effects of acupuncture on climacteric vasomotor symptoms, quality of life, and urinary excretion of neuropeptides among postmenopausal women. *Menopause* 1995; **2**: 3–12.

26. Hammar M, Berg G, Lindgren R. Does physical exercise influence the frequency of postmenopausal hot flushes? *Acta Obstet Gynecol Scand* 1991; **69**: 409–12.

27. Coope J, Thomson JM, Poller L. Effects of 'natural oestrogen' replacement therapy on menopausal symptoms and blood clotting. *BMJ* 1975; **4**: 139–43.

28. Sherwin BB, Gelfand MM. A prospective one-year study of estrogen and progestin in postmenopausal women: effects on clinical symptoms and lipoprotein lipids. *Obstet Gynecol* 1989; **73**: 759–66.

29. Notelovitz M, Arce J-C, Nanavati N, Huang WC. Norethindrone acetate at 0.5 mg dose adds to the efficacy of 1 mg 17β-estradiol on vasomotor symptom relief. *Menopause* 1998; **5**: 250–1.

30. Schiff I, Tulchinsky D, Cramer D, Ryan KJ. Oral medroxyprogesterone in the treatment of

postmenopausal symptoms. *JAMA* 1980; **244**: 1443–5.

31. Clayden JR, Bell JW, Pollard P. Menopausal flushing: double-blind trial of a non-hormonal medication. *BMJ* 1975; **1**: 409–12.

32. Jones KP, Ravnikar V, Schiff I. A preliminary evaluation of the effect of lofexidine on vasomotor flushes in post-menopausal women. *Maturitas* 1985; 7: 135–9.

33. Nesheim B-I, Saetre T. Reduction of menopausal hot flushes by methyldopa: a double blind crossover trial. *Eur J Clin Pharmacol* 1981; **20**: 413–16.

34. Lebherz TB, French L. Nonhormonal treatment of the menopausal syndrome. *Obstet Gynecol* 1969; **33**: 795–9.

35. Melis GB, Gambacciani M, Cagnacci A et al. Effects of the dopamine antagonist veralipride on hot flushes and luteinizing hormone secretion in postmenopausal women. *Obstet Gynecol* 1988; **72**: 688–92.

36. Coope J, Williams S, Patterson JS. A study of the effectiveness of propranolol in menopausal hot flushes. *Br J Obstet Gynaecol* 1978; **85**: 472–5.

37. Alcoff JM, Campbell D, Tribble D et al. Double-blind, placebo-controlled, crossover trial of propranolol as treatment for menopausal vasomotor symptoms. *Clin Ther* 1981; **3**: 356–64.

38. Albertazzi P, Pansini F, Bonaccorsi G et al. The effect of dietary soy supplementation of hot flushes. *Obstet Gynecol* 1998; **91**: 6–11.

39. Dalais FS, Rice GE, Wahlqvist ML et al. Effects of dietary phytoestrogens in postmenopausal women. *Climacteric* 1998; **1**: 124–9.

40. Stoll W. Phytotherapeutikum beeinflußt atrophisches Vaginalepithel – Doppelblindversuch Cimicifuga vs Östrogenpräparat. *Therapeutikon* 1985; **1**: 1–15.

41. Liske E, Wüstenberg P. Therapy of climacteric complaints with *Cimicifuga racemosa*: herbal medicine with clinically proven evidence. *Menopause* 1998; **5**: 250 [abstract].

42. Fisher B, Costantino J, Wickerham DL et al for the National Surgical Adjuvant Breast and Bowel Project Investigators. Tamoxifen for prevention of breast cancer: report of the National Surgical Adjuvant Breast and Bowel Project P-1 Study. *J Natl Cancer Inst* 1998; **90**: 1371–88.

43. Draper MW, Flower DE, Huster WJ et al. A controlled trial of raloxifene (LY 139481) HCL: impact on bone turnover and serum lipid profile in healthy postmenopausal women. *J Bone Miner Res* 1996; **11**: 835–42.

44. Walsh BW, Kuller LH, Wild RA et al. Effects of raloxifene on serum lipids and coagulation factors in healthy postmenopausal women. *JAMA* 1998; **279**: 1445–51.

45. Delmas PD, Bjarnason NH, Mitlak BH et al. Effects of raloxifene on bone mineral density, serum cholesterol concentrations, and uterine endometrium in postmenopausal women. *N Engl J Med* 1997; **337**: 1641–7.

46. Cummings SR, Eckert S, Krueger KA et al. The effect of raloxifene on risk of breast cancer in post-menopausal women. *JAMA* 1999; **281**: 2189–97.

47. Davies GC, Huster WJ, Lu Y et al. Adverse events reported by postmenopausal women in controlled trials with raloxifene. *Obstet Gynecol* 1999; **93**: 558–65.

48. Baker VL, Draper M, Paul S et al. Reproductive endocrine and endometrial effects of raloxifene hydrochloride, a selective

estrogen receptor modulator, in women with regular menstrual cycles. *J Clin Endocrinol Metab* 1998; **83**: 6–13.

49. Merchenthaler I, Funkhouser JM, Carver JM et al. Effect of estrogens and antiestrogens in a rat model for hot flush. *Maturitas* 1998; **30**: 307–16.

50. Bolognese M, Moffett A, Jensen C, MacDonald B. Idoxifene is well tolerated in osteopenic postmenopausal women. *Menopause* 1998; **5**: 271–2 [abstract].

51. Toran-Allerand CD. Interactions of estrogen with growth factors in the developing central nervous system. In: Hochberg RB, Naftolin F (eds). *The New Biology of Steroid Hormones.* Raven Press: New York, 1994: 311–24.

52. Haskell SG, Richardson ED, Horwitz RI. The effect of estrogen replacement therapy on cognitive function in women: a critical review of the literature. *J Clin Epidemiol* 1997; **50**: 1249–64.

53. Yaffe K, Sawaya G, Lieberburg I, Grady D. Estrogen therapy in postmenopausal women. Effects on cognitive function and dementia. *JAMA* 1998; **279**: 688–95.

54. Polo-Kantola P, Portin R, Koskinen T et al. Climacteric symptoms do not impair cognitive performances in postmenopause. *Maturitas* 1997; **27**: 13–23.

55. Reboussin BA, Greendale G, Espeland MA. Effect of hormone replacement therapy on self-reported cognitive symptoms: results from the Postmenopausal Estrogen/Progestin Interventions (PEPI) trial. *Climacteric* 1998; **1**: 172–9.

56. Nickelsen T, Lufkin EG, Riggs BL et al. Raloxifene hydrochloride, a selective estrogen receptor modulator: safety assessment of effects on cognitive function and mood in postmenopausal women. *Psychoneuroendocrinology* 1999; **24**: 115–23.

57. Nilsen J, Mor G, Naftolin F. Raloxifene induces neurite outgrowth in estrogen receptor positive PC12 cells. *Menopause* 1998; **5**: 211–16.

58. Siefer DB, Roa-Pena L, Keefe DL et al. Increasing hypothalamic arcuate nucleus glial peroxidase activity in ageing female rats is reduced by an antiestrogen and a gonadotropin-releasing hormone agonist. *Menopause* 1994; **1**: 83–90.

59. Clemens JA, Bennett DR, Black LJ, Jones CD. Effects of a new antiestrogen, keoxifene (LY156758), on growth of carcinogen-induced mammary tumors and on LH and prolaction levels. *Life Sci* 1983; **32**: 2869–75.

60. Shugrue PJ, Lane MV, Merchenthaler I. Regulation of progesterone receptor messenger ribonucleic acid in the rat medial preoptic nucleus by estrogenic and antiestrogenic compounds: an in situ hybridization study. *Endocrinology* 1997; **138**: 5476–84.

61. Collins A, Landgren B-M. Reproductive health use of estrogen and experience of symptoms in perimenopausal women: a population-based study. *Maturitas* 1994; **20**: 101–11.

62. Dennerstein L, Smith AMA, Morse C. Psychological well-being, mid-life and the menopause. *Maturitas* 1994; **20**: 1–11.

63. Kaufert P, Gilbert P, Tate R. The Manitoba project: a re-examining of the link between menopause and depression. *Maturitas* 1992; **14**: 143–56.

64. Limouzin-Lamothe MA, Mairin N, Joyce CR, Le-Gal M. Quality of life after the menopause: influence of hormonal replacement therapy. *Am J Obstet Gynecol* 1994; **170**: 618–24.

65. Zweifel JE, O'Brien WH. A meta-analysis of

the effect of hormone replacement therapy upon depressed mood. *Psychoneuroendocrinology* 1997; **22**: 189–212.

66. Daly E, Gray A, Barlow D et al. Measuring the impact of menopausal symptoms on quality of life. *BMJ* 1993; **307**: 836–40.

67. Groeneveld FPMJ, Bareman FP, Barentsen R et al. Vasomotor symptoms and well-being in the climacteric years. *Maturitas* 1996; **23**: 293–9.

68. Holte A. Menopause, mood and hormone replacement therapy: methodological issues. *Maturitas* 1998; **29**: 5–18.

69. Palinkas LA, Barrett-Connor E. Estrogen use and depressive symptoms in postmenopausal women. *Obstet Gynecol* 1992; **80**: 30–6.

70. McCoy NL. Methodological problems in the study of sexuality and the menopause. *Maturitas* 1998; **29**: 51–60.

71. Sherwin BB. The use of androgens in the postmenopause: evidence from clinical studies. In: Wren BG (ed). *Progress in the Management of the Menopause.* Parthenon Publishing: Lancaster, 1997: 263–6.

72. Samsioe G, Heraib F, Lidfeldt J et al. Urogenital symptoms in women aged 50–60. *Gynecol Endocrinol* 1999; **13**: 113–7.

73. Dören M. Urogenital aging – creation of improved awareness. *Am J Obstet Gynecol* 1998; **178**: S254–6.

74. Fantl JA, Cardozo LA, McClish DK and the Hormones and the Urogenital Therapy Committee. Estrogen therapy in the management of urinary incontinence in postmenopausal women: a meta-analysis. First report of the Hormones and Urogenital Therapy Committee. *Obstet Gynecol* 1994; **83**: 112–18.

75. Sultana CJ, Walters MD. Estrogen and urinary incontinence. *Maturitas* 1994; **20**: 129–38.

76. Barlow DH, Samsioe G, van Geelen JM. A study of European women's experience of the problems of urogenital ageing and its management. *Maturitas* 1997; **27**: 239–47.

77. Thom DH, Brown JS. Reproductive and hormonal risk factors for urinary incontinence in later life: a review of the clinical and epidemiologic literature. *J Am Geriatr Soc* 1998; **46**: 1411–17.

78. Cardozo L, Bachmann G, McClish D et al. Meta-analysis of estrogen therapy in the management of urogenital atrophy in postmenopausal women: Second Report of the Hormones and Urogenital Therapy Committee. *Obstet Gynecol* 1998; **92**: 722–7.

8

The effect of SERMs on the reproductive system

Patrick Neven

There is experimental and clinical evidence that raloxifene differs from tamoxifen and oestrogen with respect to its long-term endometrial effect. In the uterus, raloxifene acts by a different mechanism to that of classical oestrogens and tamoxifen. Uterine safety with raloxifene is based on reliable data from a large number of patients treated for 3 years.

Introduction

Selective oestrogen receptor modulators (SERMs) comprise a group of structurally diverse compounds that are distinguished from oestrogens by their ability to interact with the oestrogen receptor (ER) and to act as either a pure oestrogen agonist, a partial agonist or an oestrogen antagonist. The net effect depends on the species studied, the target organ examined, the endpoint measured, treatment dose and duration, and endogenous oestrogen levels. There are a number of synthetic compounds that display a mixed oestrogen agonist/antagonist profile. The best known and considered as the first generation of SERMs are the triphenylethylenes, such as tamoxifen, toremifene, droloxifene and idoxifene. The second generation of SERMs have a different chemical structure. They include benzothiophene derivatives, such as raloxifene.

An assessment of endometrial safety is mandatory for any compound containing an active substance able to bind to the ER. This chapter describes the effect of the different SERMs on the reproductive system; most attention is given to their uterine effects but potential actions on the cervix, vagina and ovary are also considered.

The clinical importance of SERMs

Oestrogen is an ambivalent steroid hormone. On the one hand, it protects postmenopausal women against osteoporosis, cardiovascular disease, vaginal dryness and tooth loss, and probably against many other degenerative conditions such as skin changes, Alzheimer's disease and related neurodegenerative dementias. On the other hand, oestrogen is implicated in the development of breast and uterine cancers. In 1896, Beatson[1] observed that bilateral oophorectomy was effective in advanced breast cancer in premenopausal women and in 1927 Murray[2] showed that transplantation of the ovary to male rodents caused cancer in the male breast. Nowadays, all endocrine therapies for breast cancer are designed to reduce serum oestrogen levels or to block the effects of oestrogens on cancer cells. They are successfully used to improve the disease-free survival of breast cancer patients and are today's major treatment modality for the management of breast cancer.[3]

Most of the risk factors that have been linked to endometrial cancer have also been associated with excessive oestrogen. Long exposure to endogenous oestrogen, such as in women with an early menarche, late menopause, regular non-interrupted menstrual cycles (nulliparity), chronic anovulation and obesity, increases a woman's risk of endometrial cancer. Pregnancy and the combined oral contraceptive pill confer protection from endometrial carcinoma by interrupting the continued stimulation of the endometrium by oestrogens. Case–control and cohort studies have demonstrated an increase in the relative risk (RR) for endometrial cancer associated with unopposed oestrogen use for menopausal symptoms.[4] The RR is positively correlated to the dose and duration of exposure, ranging from two- to ninefold. The histological changes seen in patients treated with oestrogen and combined oestrogen, with less than 12 days of recommended progestin combinations, encompass a variety of patterns leading to endometrial hyperplasia and cancer.[5] Even continuous combined oestro-progestogens, which increase patient compliance by eliminating withdrawal bleeding, have recently been associated with an increased endometrial cancer risk.[6] The issue of ensuring endometrial safety by adding progestins to continuous oestrogen replacement is still under debate.

The search for the ideal oestrogen, which mimics the beneficial effects of oestrogen and/or blocks the adverse ones, has been going on for almost half a century.

Diethylstilbestrol, a non-steroidal compound and synthesized in 1938, was the first SERM. It mimics the effects of oestrogens; bone mineral density increases and in the long term endometrial cancer risk increases. High doses are antioestrogenic and effective in advanced breast cancer. Successive chemical modifications of the oestrogenic stilbene nucleus of diethylstilbestrol, driven by their anticipated application as antioestrogens for oral contraception, led, in the 1940s and 1950s, to the development of a class of non-toxic molecules with antioestrogenic properties called the triphenylethylenes. Although antifertile in the rat, the triphenylethylenes had the opposite effect in premenopausal women, causing ovarian steroidogenesis and ovulation induction. Clomiphene is an example of a triphenylethylene still used as a fertility agent.

The second focus of these new antioestrogenic compounds was for use in breast cancer, which is often oestrogen-dependent. The triphenylethylene derivative, tamoxifen, developed by Imperial Chemical Industries (ICI; UK) in 1966 is still the most widely used and studied SERM. At about the same time that Toft and Gorski discovered the existence of the ER in some breast cancers as a possible biochemical marker for oestrogen dependency,[7] ICI launched their first tamoxifen trials in women with metastatic ER-positive breast cancer. More than 30 years and ten million women-years later, tamoxifen has become the endocrine treatment of choice for all stages of breast cancer, especially in postmenopausal women with ER-positive tumours. The worldwide overview on tamoxifen as an adjuvant for breast cancer therapy from the Early Breast Cancer Trialists' Collaborative Group published in 1998 showed that tamoxifen treatment in postmenopausal women reduced mortality by almost 25% and reduced the recurrence of breast cancer by 50%.[3] Because of its very low toxicity, today's general recommendation is to prescribe 20 mg tamoxifen daily for 5 years. Whether longer term treatment is better is still under consideration.

Tamoxifen has a SERM profile with tissue-specific oestrogenic and antioestrogenic properties. While it is antioestrogenic in the breast, in other tissues it has oestrogen agonist properties, for example in the uterus and bone, probably because these tissues have proteins that augment transcription via one of the binding regions of the ER. The exact molecular basis for its contradictory profile of biological effects is not known but seems to derive from divergent intracellular signalling pathways and target genes. The ER protein is

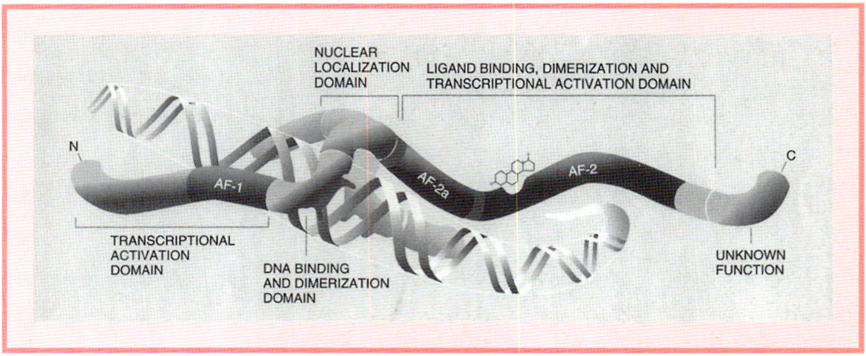

Figure 8.1
The oestrogen receptor protein. (Illustration by Anne Erickson. Reproduced from ref. 8.)

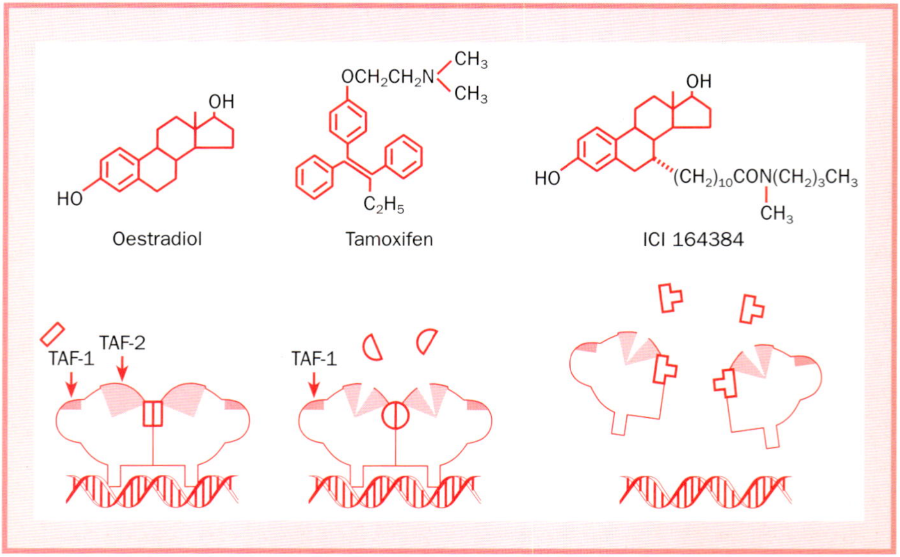

Figure 8.2
Model for the action of oestrogen, tamoxifen and ICI 164,384 on the oestrogen receptor. (Reproduced from ref. 9.)

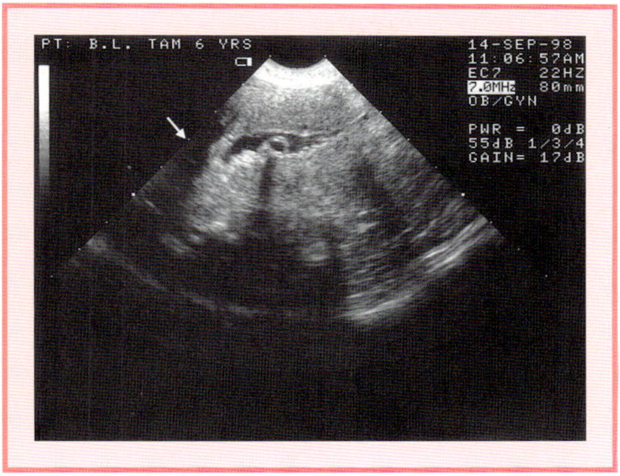

Figure 8.3
Saline infusion sonography of a tamoxifen-thickened pseudopolypoid glandulocystic endometrium.

a transcription factor that is composed of several regions responsible for specific functions (***Figure 8.1***). A hypothetical model to explain tamoxifen's oestrogenic/ antioestrogenic activities has been designed and is shown in ***Figure 8.2***.[9] Following ER binding, both oestradiol and tamoxifen lead to DNA activation through the constitutively active transcription activation factor (AF-1); this explains its oestrogenic effect. Tamoxifen, however, competes with oestradiol for the same ER-binding place, preventing activation of AF-2 and causing an antioestrogenic effect.

The oestrogenic action of tamoxifen in reducing osteoporotic fractures[10] and myocardial infarction[11] amongst postmenopausal women has stimulated current trials to explore the use of tamoxifen as a breast cancer prophylactic agent in healthy women. Currently, thousands of healthy women in the USA, Europe and Australia are participating in such trials. In the placebo-controlled trial from the USA (NSABP-P1), with an average follow-up of 3.6 years, tamoxifen reduced ER-positive breast cancer risk in all age groups by 45%; this effect increased with age (35% < 49 years versus 53% > 60 years) and with a longer duration of tamoxifen treatment.[12] The beneficial effects of tamoxifen for breast cancer prevention were not confirmed by the Royal Marsden tamoxifen chemoprevention trial[13] or the Italian Tamoxifen Prevention

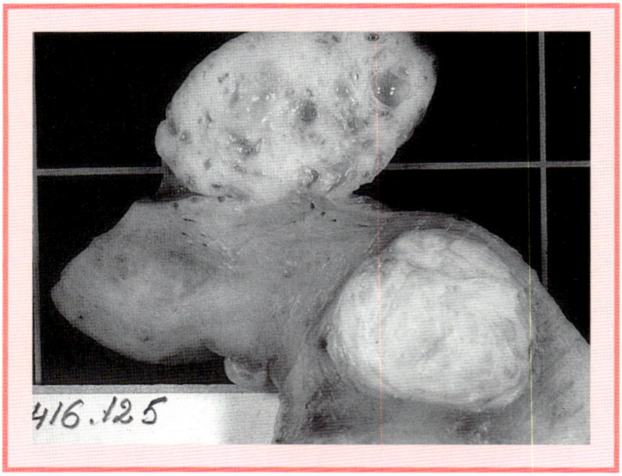

Figure 8.4
Histopathologic image of a glandulocystic polyp cancer and intramural fibroid.

Study.[14] The trials, however, were smaller and enrolled lower risk women than did the NSABP trial.

Tamoxifen and the reproductive tract

The uterus

In premenopausal women, tamoxifen predominantly produces antioestrogenic effects in the uterus despite circulating supraphysiological oestradiol levels. In the postmenopausal patient because of its partial oestrogen agonistic activity, up to 30% of women taking tamoxifen have gynaecological problems; abnormal vaginal bleeding and discharge are most often reported. A number of asymptomatic endometrial changes, mainly stromal fibrosis leading to cystic dilated endometrial glands (***Figure 8.3***), appear as early as 6 months following treatment with tamoxifen; such changes are easily seen using transvaginal ultrasonography (TVU). Tamoxifen may also cause proliferative and neoplastic uterine lesions such as endometrial hyperplasia, polyposis, fibroid growth, carcinoma and sarcomas. Adenomyosis, probably induced de novo, and reactivation of dormant/de novo endometriosis have both been reported in postmenopausal women on tamoxifen.[15]

Increasing attention has been paid to the relationship between tamoxifen and endometrial changes. Postmenopausal breast cancer patients on 20 mg tamoxifen daily more often have a high incidence of benign

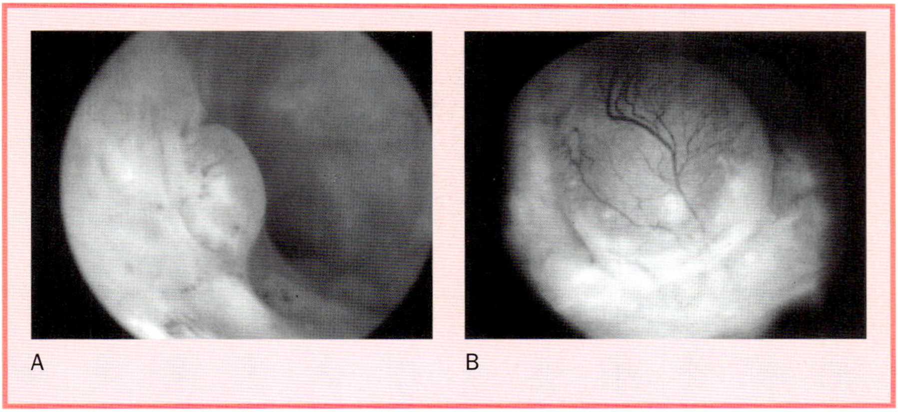

Figure 8.5
Hysteroscopic images of tamoxifen-induced pseudopolypoid glandulocystic endometrium.

endometrial and endocervical polyps and of hyperplastic endometrial layer than do a matched control group of breast cancer patients, independent of whether or not they report postmenopausal vaginal bleeding.[16] In a population of postmenopausal patients starting with a thin rectilinear endometrium, as detected by TVU, tamoxifen's oestrogen-like activity leads to the occurrence of endometrial abnormalities in over 50% of cases, even within the first year of treatment. Once the endometrium becomes thickened, the positive predictive value and specificity of TVU are very poor. Ultrasound cannot differentiate between the potentially dangerous glandulocystic polyp cancers (*Figure 8.4*) and the glandulocystic appearances of the endometrial stroma (*Figure 8.5*).

Tissue diagnosis is mandatory in women with a sonographically abnormal endometrium. Because blind endometrial biopsies have serious limitations in the investigation of endometrium thickening, rigorous evaluation requires saline infusion sonography (SIS) or hysteroscopy with guided endometrial biopsies. In the case of a pseudopolypoid glandulocystic endometrium there is, on hysteroscopy, a smooth white but hypervascularized endometrial layer with many scattered protuberances. These protuberances consist of a thin atrophic endometrium overlying a cystic dilated gland with an oedematous stroma. In SIS, there is an empty cavity with a Gruyère cheese appearance of the subepithelial layer of the endometrium. Histologically, this

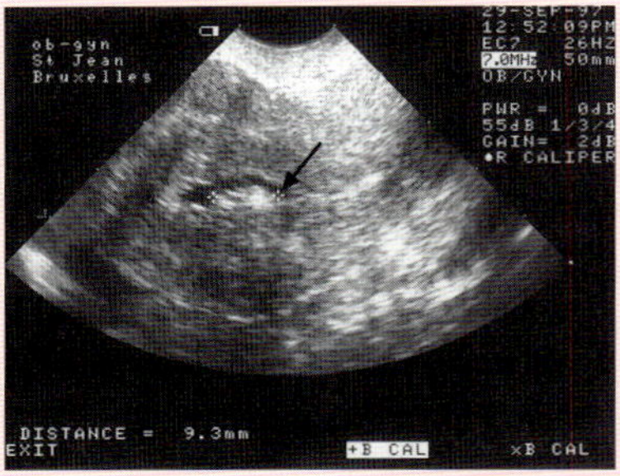

Figure 8.6
SIS image of tamoxifen-induced glandulocystic polyp.

endometrium typically shows periglandular stromal condensation, epithelial metaplasia and proliferative activity, sometimes with varying degrees of cytological atypia. In the case of a polyp, SIS reveals a glandulocystic structure which is free floating and surrounded with saline (*Figure 8.6*); on hysteroscopy, the endometrium surrounding the polyp is mostly thick and irregular. The majority of endometrial polyps occur on a background of simple endometrial hyperplasia; however, the neighbouring endometrium may be atrophic. Microscopically, the polyps are characterized by patchy periglandular condensation of stroma, proliferative activity in epithelial and stromal cells and an admixture of epithelial metaplasias, including squamoid and mucinous metaplasias. It is highly unusual for these three microscopic features to coexist in the same polyp in women not using tamoxifen.[17]

More than 300 cases of endometrial cancer have been related to tamoxifen in postmenopausal women undergoing treatment for breast cancer. Breast and endometrial cancers share common risk factors and evidence exists that some endometrial cancers in patients taking tamoxifen were present before the women started taking the drug or were related to other risk factors such as obesity or previous oestrogen replacement therapy. However, three well-designed studies adequately controlling for background risks clearly show a carcinogenic effect of tamoxifen on the human endometrium.[18–20] These three trials were large studies of postmenopausal women with follow-up times of at least 4.5 years. In our own literature review, using all reported endometrial cancers from placebo-controlled trials with tamoxifen, we found a twofold increase in the incidence rate of endometrial carcinoma risk in tamoxifen-treated patients (0.79% versus 0.37%).[21] There seems to be an increasing risk with total dose and duration of intake but the biological behaviour of endometrial cancers from tamoxifen is not different from those developing in women not on tamoxifen. Tamoxifen is now classified by the International Agency for Research on Cancer as a human endometrial carcinogen.[22] Although most clinicians agree that long-term tamoxifen users have an increased risk of endometrial cancer, this risk should not be overestimated and does not alter the risk–benefit ratio for breast cancer patients on tamoxifen.

Tamoxifen's endometrial effect appears similar in healthy postmenopausal women. In one such population, assigned to receive either tamoxifen or placebo with a mean follow-up time of 22 months, histological evidence of an abnormal endometrium was found in 39% of the tamoxifen group and 10% of the control group, although all changes were benign.[23] In the NSABP-P1 study, where a close to normal postmenopausal population participated in a tamoxifen versus placebo-controlled breast cancer chemoprevention trial, tamoxifen intake was associated with a 2.5-fold excess risk of endometrial carcinoma.[12] This is the first report in the literature of patients without breast cancer who received tamoxifen and developed endometrial cancer; this increased risk of endometrial cancer in healthy women taking tamoxifen has caused concern about the safety of long-term tamoxifen treatment. This potential side effect is especially important for the large groups of healthy women exposed to the antioestrogen tamoxifen for the prevention of breast cancer.

Other parts of the reproductive tract

In premenopausal women, tamoxifen stimulates ovarian steroidogenesis and induces a two- to threefold sustained increase in circulating oestradiol levels without intermediary gonadotrophin stimulation. The levels of follicle-stimulating hormone (FSH) and luteinizing hormone (LH) remain in the normal range; progesterone is elevated and prolactin falls. The relative increase in total oestrogens is higher than can be accommodated by the rise in sex hormone binding globulin. This leads to an increase in the urinary excretion of total oestrogens, reflecting a rise in the concentration of circulating biologically available oestrogens. Irregular cycles are common during tamoxifen treatment and amenorrhoea may occur in up to 25%. In treated premenopausal women 10% may also have ovarian cysts, and complications with these cysts may require surgical intervention.

In postmenopausal women, circulating levels of oestradiol and progesterone are low and tamoxifen does not cause an elevation in circulating oestrogens. It lowers serum gonadotrophin levels, although these remain within the normal postmenopausal range. There is no evidence that tamoxifen induces ovarian cysts in postmenopausal patients. Extensive clinical use of tamoxifen in pre- and postmenopausal women has not been associated with an increased risk of ovarian cancer. Tamoxifen has been used in women with advanced ovarian cancers; responses have been reported but rates are low.

In contrast with tamoxifen's atrophic effect on the vagina in premenopausal women, most authors agree that in 50% of postmenopausal women tamoxifen has an oestrogen agonist effect on the vaginal epithelium. One in five postmenopausal women noted an increase in vaginal discharge.

Focus on raloxifene

The ability of tamoxifen to evoke a heterogeneous and often contrasting set of responses from classic oestrogen-sensitive organs signalled the feasibility of selective oestrogen antagonism/agonism and accelerated the race for the development of the 'ideal oestrogen'. Because of the unwanted uterine side effects with tamoxifen, attention has now shifted to the tamoxifen-related benzothiophenes which were also, many years ago, developed for the treatment of breast cancer. The most extensively researched has been raloxifene. Like tamoxifen, raloxifene evokes differential oestrogenic (e.g. bone) or antioestrogenic (e.g. breast) responses. In contrast with tamoxifen, raloxifene seems neutral with respect to endometrial activity. The growth stimulatory effects of oestrogens and the antioestrogens, tamoxifen and raloxifene, have been examined at a molecular level in vitro and in vivo. An ER-positive endometrial cancer cell line grew when it was treated with tamoxifen and oestradiol. Raloxifene behaved in these cells as an antioestrogen and inhibited oestradiol and tamoxifen-induced growth (***Figure 8.7***); in contrast with oestradiol and tamoxifen, raloxifene had no effect on insulin growth factor binding protein release.[24] In ovariectomized rats, oestradiol and tamoxifen increased the mitotic activity and progesterone receptor synthesis of luminal epithelial cells of the endometrium, but raloxifene was much less effective. Raloxifene caused a slight increase in uterine wet weight and endometrial stromal thickness but, in contrast with the effect of tamoxifen, stromal eosinophilia was not seen; the endometrium did not proliferate and there was no dose response over the dosage range tested.[25] Another experimental study has shown that raloxifene inhibits tamoxifen-induced endometrial proliferation in ovariectomized rats.[26] The uterine effect of raloxifene in ovariectomized cynomolgus monkeys showed dose-dependent uterine atrophy.

Although SERMs interact through the same ER as oestradiol, the net endometrial response differs from that of oestradiol and between different SERMs. The exact molecular mechanisms behind oestradiol/raloxifene/tamoxifen's uterotrophic activity and the uterine cellular compartments that respond to the drugs have not been clearly established. However, there is

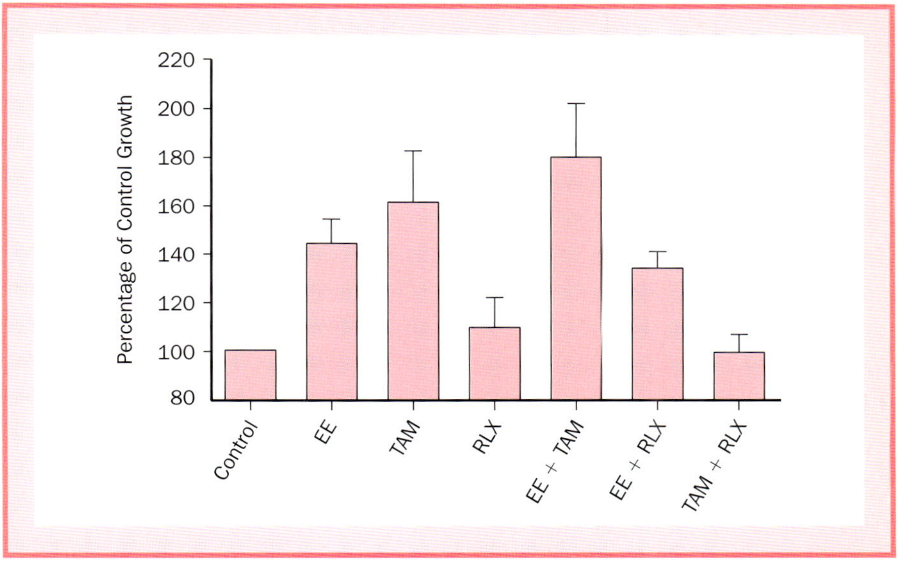

Figure 8.7
Raloxifene inhibits endometrial cancer cell proliferation.

experimental evidence that although the oestradiol/tamoxifen–ER complex binds to the oestrogen response element, in uterine tissues it can also bind to DNA sites that do not contain oestrogen response elements, for example the AP-1 site on oestrogen-sensitive target genes. It is believed that both oestradiol and tamoxifen act through the AP-1 site in uterine tissue but that raloxifene does not, which may explain why raloxifene has a different endometrial effect.[27]

Another possible explanation for the tissue-dependent response is that the different actions are due to the existence of two ERs and the tissue-dependent expression of ERα and ERβ. A second ER (ERβ) with a unique tissue distribution and different affinities for oestrogen agonists and antagonists has recently been described.[28] With ERα, oestradiol activates transcription from the AP-1 site whereas with ERβ oestradiol inhibits transcription.[29] Whereas the action of oestradiol and tamoxifen is mediated through the activation of ERα, raloxifene may preferentially bind the ERβ. Such differences in ligand activity, together with the different distributions of the two receptors in the body, may help to explain oestrogen's broad spectrum of activity and some of the paradoxical effects of antioestrogens.

Raloxifene and the reproductive tract

The uterus

In healthy postmenopausal women, several double-blind, placebo-controlled studies evaluated the effects of raloxifene on the uterus. Whereas in the past, blind endometrial biopsies were the most commonly employed endometrial sampling technique, ultrasound and hysteroscopy have recently been advocated as more reliable in evaluating the uterine cavity. Uterine safety in raloxifene studies was assessed from evaluation of endometrial biopsies, transvaginal endometrial ultrasound (TVU), SIS, hysteroscopy and the incidence of postmenopausal bleeding.

In an 8-week randomized, double-blind, placebo-controlled, multicentre Phase II study, 251 healthy postmenopausal women received 0.625 mg/day conjugated equine oestrogens or 200 or 600 mg/day raloxifene. Treatment with raloxifene did not induce histopathologic evidence of endometrial stimulation in healthy postmenopausal women, as assessed by an oestrogenicity scoring system.[30]

In an osteoporosis preventive study, the effect of placebo and 30, 60, or 150 mg of raloxifene on endometrial thickness (ET) was studied in 444 women.[31] In the raloxifene prevention trials, TVU was used to assess ET every 6 months for the first 2 years and then annually thereafter. If the ET was more than 5 mm after retest or if bleeding occurred, with or without increased ET, or if, in the investigator's opinion, biopsy was otherwise warranted, the uterine cavity was assessed by SIS or hysteroscopy and an endometrial sample was obtained by Pipelle biopsy. This study indicates that raloxifene intake for 2 years does not lead to uterine or endometrial stimulation (***Figure 8.8***). Preliminary results from the third-year analysis indicate no change in endometrial thickness during raloxifene therapy. Likewise, vaginal bleeding was rarely reported by raloxifene or placebo-treated subjects during the first 2 years of therapy, with no difference in the incidence between treatment and placebo groups. Again, this has not changed during 3 years of therapy. Recently, data from 1157 postmenopausal women on raloxifene 60 mg daily were analyzed for vaginal bleeding and increased endometrial thickness. For up to 30 months, raloxifene is not associated with vaginal bleeding or endometrial thickening in postmenopausal women.

In another ongoing study, a long-term comparison of 150 mg raloxifene versus continuous conjugated oestrogens and medroxyprogesterone acetate, the effects on

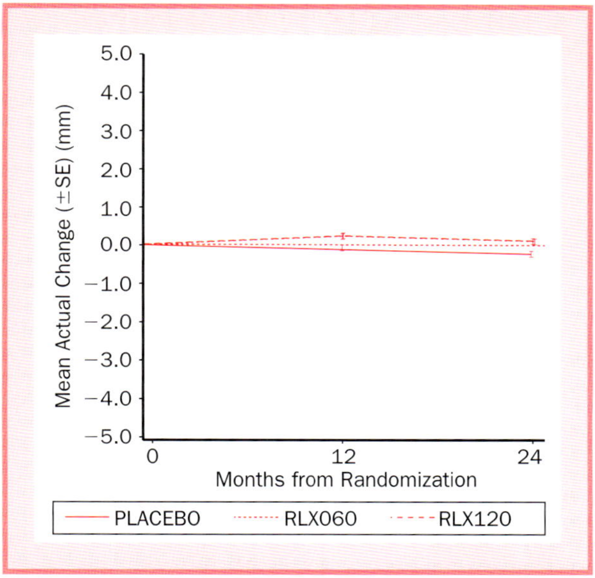

Figure 8.8
Changes in endometrial thickness by treatment. Mean with one standard error.

the uterus in postmenopausal women were evaluated.[33] The study compared the effects of each therapy on endometrial thickness, uterine volume, histologic characteristics and bleeding. At baseline, proliferative endometrium was present in 4.3% of women treated with 150 mg raloxifene versus 2.6% of hormone replacement therapy (HRT)-treated women. An interim analysis of 12-month data from this 2-year study found that raloxifene does not have undesirable stimulatory effects on the uterus. Mean endometrial thickness for the HRT group increased by 0.62 mm, a statistically significant increase over baseline ($p = 0.017$), whereas the mean increase of 0.18 mm noted for the raloxifene group was not statistically significant. Mean uterine volume for the HRT group increased by 21.2 ml, which was a significant change from baseline ($p < 0.001$). In contrast, the raloxifene group had a decrease of 3 ml in mean uterine volume, a change that was not statistically significant. Biopsies revealed no endometrial hyperplasia in either group. At the endpoint a proliferative endometrium developed in 31.6% of subjects in the HRT group versus 2.2% in the raloxifene group. In 9% of the women on continuous HRT, vaginal bleeding led to discontinuation while in the raloxifene group there was no discontinuation as a result of vaginal bleeding. Furthermore, the raloxifene group showed a significantly lower oestrogenicity grade at endpoint compared with the HRT group ($p = 0.020$). These results demonstrate that even at 1 year, raloxifene clearly does not have tamoxifen-like effects, with virtually no hyperplasia or polyp formation compared with the previously stated incidence rate of 18% hyperplasia and 25–30% polyp formation reported with tamoxifen. Considering all randomized trials with raloxifene, uterine-related adverse events were analysed for almost 6000 postmenopausal women who had not had a prior hysterectomy. There were no statistically significant treatment group differences with respect to adverse events related to vaginal bleeding.

Using all endometrial cancer cases reported in women participating in all placebo-controlled trials with raloxifene, although based on a small number of cases, it seems that raloxifene decreased the endometrial cancer incidence by more than half (RR = 0.38).[34] In the MORE trial, raloxifene did not increase the risk of endometrial cancer during the first three years (RR = 0.67), but the total number of cases was small.[35] These data suggest that a possible effect of raloxifene may be to decrease the rate of incident endometrial carcinoma.

Other parts of the reproductive tract

Clinical trials with raloxifene in postmenopausal women have, after 39 months of exposure, produced no evidence of cervical problems, ovarian abnormalities or increased ovarian cancer risk as recently seen with hormone replacement therapy.[36] Serum gonadotrophins are not increased in postmenopausal women on raloxifene.

Preliminary results suggest that raloxifene has no effect on the vaginal mucosa; neither dyspareunia nor urinary frequency were reported more frequently as adverse events in those women using raloxifene.

Other antioestrogens

In the animal model, droloxifene had a lower oestrogenic and a higher antioestrogenic effect on the uterine weight of rats than tamoxifen. Idoxifene is an approximately 10-fold less potent antioestrogen in immature rat uterine weight tests. However, it has less uterotropic activity when administered alone. Trials with droloxifene and idoxifene have been withdrawn because neither SERM is better than tamoxifen for breast cancer, and because of their effects on the human endometrium. Phase III trials for levormeloxifene, another SERM tested in osteoporosis treatment and prevention, were recently discontinued following observations of increased endometrial thickness, an increased frequency of urinary incontinence and utero-vaginal prolapse. Toremifene, another tamoxifen analogue approved for breast cancer treatment, is less oestrogenic at equimolar doses in the rat uterus and believed to be less carcinogenic than tamoxifen in the rat liver. Endometrial stimulation, however, has been reported in women taking toremifene.[37]

New compounds are being studied. Replacement of raloxifene's carbonyl group with oxygen, for example, resulted in a substantial (10-fold) increase in oestrogen antagonist potency relative to raloxifene. In the uterine model, it produced an even greater inhibition of uterine proliferation induced by exogenous oestrogen than raloxifene, with similar oestrogen-like effects on bone and lipids.[38]

Conclusion

SERMs are agents that, depending upon the tissue type, produce either oestrogen agonist or oestrogen antagonist activities. Tamoxifen and raloxifene produce oestrogen-like effects on bone and cholesterol metabolism and are both oestrogen antagonists in mammary tissue.

However, in the uterus, raloxifene and tamoxifen differ in their pharmacological profiles; tamoxifen behaves as a partial oestrogen agonist whereas raloxifene acts as a complete oestrogen antagonist. The second generation SERMs, such as raloxifene, appear to have an improved safety profile and represent a potentially important alternative to chronic hormone replacement in postmenopausal women considering prevention of osteoporosis and cardiovascular disease. Furthermore, they may protect against breast and endometrial cancer.

References

1. Beatson GT. On the treatment of inoperable cases of carcinoma of the mamma: suggestions for a new method of treatment, with illustrative cases. *Lancet* 1896; **ii:** 104–7, 162–5.
2. Murray WS. Ovarian secretion and tumor incidence. *Science* 1927; **66:** 600–1.
3. Early Breast Cancer Trialists' Collaborative Group. Tamoxifen for early breast cancer: an overview of the randomised trials. *Lancet* 1998; **351:** 1451–67.
4. Meissner WA, Sommers SC, Sherman BM. Endometrial hyperplasia, endometrial carcinoma and endometriose produced experimentally by estrogen. *Cancer* 1957; **10:** 500–9.
5. Beresford SAA, Weiss NS, Voigt L, McKnight B. Risk of endometrial cancer in relation to oestrogen combined with cyclic progestogen therapy in postmenopausal women. *Lancet* 1997; **349:** 458–61.
6. Comerci JT, Goldberg GL, Runowicz CD, Fields AL. Continuous low dose combined hormone replacement therapy and the risk of endometrial cancer. *Gynecol Oncol* 1997; **64:** 425–30.

7. Toft D, Gorski J. A receptor molecule for estrogens: isolation from the rat uterus and preliminary characterisation. *Proc Natl Acad Sci U S A* 1966; **55**: 1574–81.

8. Osborne CK. Elledge RM, Fuqua SAW. Estrogen receptors in breast cancer therapy. *Sci Am Sci Med* 1996; **3**: 32–41.

9. Parker MG, Fawell SE, Lees JA et al. Function of ER as a transcription factor: a target for antiestrogens. In: Brugge J, Curran E, McCormick F (eds). *Origins of Human Cancer: A Comprehensive Review.* Cold Spring Harbour Laboratory Press: New York, 1991: 667–74.

10. Love RR, Mazess RB, Barden HS et al. Effects of tamoxifen on bone mineral density in postmenopausal women with breast cancer. *N Engl J Med* 1992; **326**: 852–6.

11. Love RR, Wiebe DA, Newcomb PA, Chappell RJ. Effects of tamoxifen on cardiovascular risk factors in postmenopausal women after 5 years of treatment. *J Natl Cancer Inst* 1994; **86**: 1534–9.

12. Fisher B, Wickerman DL, Costantino JC et al. Tamoxifen for prevention of breast cancer: report of the NSABP-P1 study. *J Natl Cancer Inst* 1998; **90**: 1371–83.

13. Powles T, Eeles R, Ashley S et al. Interim analysis of the incidence of breast cancer in the Royal Marsden Hospital tamoxifen randomised chemoprevention trial. *The Lancet* 1998; **352**: 98–101.

14. Veronesi U, Maisonneuve P, Costa A et al. Prevention of breast cancer with tamoxifen: preliminary findings from the Italian randomised trial among hysterectomised women. *The Lancet* 1998; **352**: 93–97.

15. Neven P, Vergote I. Controversies regarding tamoxifen and uterine carcinoma. *Curr Opin Obstet Gynecol* 1998; **10**: 9–14.

16. Neven P, de Muylder X, van Belle Y et al. Tamoxifen and the uterus and endometrium. *Lancet* 1989; **i**: 375–6.

17. Neven P. *The Effect of Tamoxifen on the Uterus in Postmenopausal Breast Cancer Patients.* Acta Biom Lovaniensia: Leuven University Press, Leuven, Belgium, 1998.

18. Fornander T, Cedermark B, Mattsson A et al. Adjuvant tamoxifen in early breast cancer: occurrence of new primary cancers. *Lancet* 1989; **i**: 117–20.

19. Andersson M, Storm HH, Mouridsen HT. Incidence of new primary cancers after adjuvant tamoxifen therapy and radiotherapy for early breast cancer. *J Natl Cancer Inst* 1991; **83**: 1013–17.

20. Fisher B, Constantino JP, Redmond CK et al. Endometrial cancer in tamoxifen-treated breast cancer patients: findings from the National Surgical Adjuvant Breast and Bowel Project B-14. *J Natl Cancer Inst* 1994; **86**: 527–37.

21. Assikis VJ, Neven P, Jordan VC et al. A realistic clinical perspective of tamoxifen and endometrial carcinogenesis. *Eur J Cancer* 1996; **32A**: 1464–76.

22. IARC. *IARC monographs on the evaluation of carcinogenic risks to humans,* Vol. 66. International Agency for Research on Cancer: Lyon, 1996.

23. Kedar RP, Bourne TH, Powles TJ et al. Effects of tamoxifen on uterus and ovaries of postmenopausal women in a randomized breast cancer prevention trial. *Lancet* 1994; **343**: 1318–21.

24. Kleinman D, Karas M, Danilenko M et al. Stimulation of endometrial cancer cell growth by tamoxifen is associated with an increased

insulin-like growth factor (IGF)-I induced tyrosine phosphorylation and reduction in IGF binding proteins. *Endocrinology* 1996; **137**: 1089–95.

25. Black LJ, Sato M, Rowley ER et al. Raloxifene (LY 139481 HCl) prevents bone loss and reduces serum cholesterol without causing uterine hypertrophy in ovariectomized rats. *J Clin Invest* 1994; **93**: 63–9.

26. Fuchs-Young R, Magee DE, Cole HW et al. Raloxifene is a tissue-specific anti-estrogen that blocks tamoxifen or estrogen stimulated uterotrophic effects. *Endocrinology* 1995; **136**(suppl): S57.

27. Webb P, Lopez GN, Uht RM, Kushner PJ. Tamoxifen activation of the estrogen receptor/AP-1 pathway: potential origin for the cell-specific estrogen-like effects of antiestrogens. *Mol Endocrinol* 1995; **9**: 443–56.

28. Kuiper GG, Enmark E, Pelto-Huikko M et al. Cloning of a novel receptor expressed in rat prostate and ovary. *Proc Natl Acad Sci U S A* 1996; **93**: 5925–30.

29. Paech K, Webb P, Kuiper GGJM et al. Differential ligand activation of estrogen receptors ERα and ERβ at AP1 sites. *Science* 1997; **277**: 1508–10.

30. Boss SM, Huster WJ, Neild JA et al. Effects of raloxifene hydrochloride on the endometrium of postmenopausal women. *Am J Obstet Gynecol* 1997; **177**: 1458–64.

31. Delmas PD, Bjarnason NH, Mitlak BH et al. Effects of raloxifene on bone mineral density, serum cholesterol concentrations, and uterine endometrium in postmenopausal women. *N Engl J Med* 1997; **337**: 1641–7.

32. Davies GC, Huster WJ, Shen W et al. Endometrial response to raloxifene compared with placebo, cyclical hormone replacement therapy, and unopposed estrogen in postmenopausal women. *Menopause* 1999; **6**: 188–95.

33. Goldstein SR, Scheele WH, Symanowski SM et al. Uterine safety considerations for selective estrogen receptor modulators. *Menopause* 1997; **4**: 250.

34. Cummings SR, Norton L, Eckert S et al. Raloxifene reduces the risk of breast cancer and may decrease the risk of endometrial cancer in postmenopausal women. Two-year findings from the Multiple Outcomes of Raloxifene Evaluation (MORE) trial. Proceedings of the American Society of Clinical Oncology *Proc ASCO* 1998; **17**: 3.

35. Cummings S, Eckert S, Kneger K et al. The effect of raloxifene on risk of breast cancer in postmenopausal women. *JAMA* 1999; **281**: 2189–97.

36. Garg PP, Kerlikowske K, Subak L et al. Hormone replacement therapy and the risk of epithelial ovarian carcinoma: a meta-analysis. *Obstet Gynecol* 1998; **92**: 472–9.

37. Tomas E, Kauppila A, Blanco G et al. Comparison between the effects of tamoxifen and toremifene on the uterus in postmenopausal breast cancer patients. *Gynecol Oncol* 1995; **59**: 261–6.

38. Palkowitz AD, Glasebrook AL, Thrasher KJ et al. Discovery and synthesis of a novel highly potent SERM. *J Med Chem* 1997; **40**: 1407–16.

9

Uterine and breast safety

David Purdie

Raloxifene appears to be antagonistic to the oestrogen receptor (ER) in both myometrium and endometrium and hence is not associated with endometrial proliferation or vaginal bleeding in treated patients. Similarly, raloxifene appears to be antagonistic to the oestrogen receptor in the ducts and alveoli of the breast. Symptoms such as breast swelling and mastalgia are seen no more frequently than in controls, and the incidence of non-invasive and invasive ER+ breast cancer appears to be significantly reduced – though whether by prevention or suppression is as yet unknown.

Introduction

Breast and uterine safety are vital in oestrogen replacement. Unless an agent is deemed by the general patient population to be breast safe and uterus safe, particularly with respect to the risk of malignant disease in either organ, then that agent will fail to gain general acceptance.

Raloxifene, the first of the second-generation selective

oestrogen receptor modulators (SERMs) to be licensed, may be prescribed for the prevention of osteoporotic fracture in postmenopausal women.[1] It has no place in the treatment of premenopausal women and therefore it is in the context of the postmenopausal breast and uterus that its safety must be adjudged. The selectivity inherent in the name of these agents reflects their ability to engage the oestrogen receptor (ER) at all sites but to cause oestrogen agonism at certain sites such as the skeletal and cardiovascular systems while acting as antagonists at locations particularly within the reproductive system, such as breast and uterus, where oestrogenic activity is unwanted.

Had the oestrogens retained only their central role in preparing the maternal organism for ovulation, implantation, gestation and lactation, then the menopause, with its order of magnitude fall in the plasma concentration of oestradiol, would be of little consequence. However, these steroids have proved to be so useful for information transmission and, with their receptor, for signal transduction that they have found extra-reproductive roles (described elsewhere in this book) which may necessitate postmenopausal replacement. And therein lies the problem. The early days, indeed decades, of hormone replacement therapy (HRT) have seen major problems with patient acceptability, largely due to the re-engagement by the exogenous HRT of the ER in breast and uterus. Published studies repeatedly cite endometrial bleeding and breast complications including enlargement, tenderness and fear of breast cancer as the prime reasons why many women rejected the initiation or the continuation of HRT.[2] It had long been known that the principal cancer of the uterine corpus was adenocarcinoma, a tumour whose epidemiological risk factors such as early menarche, late menopause and obesity indicated that cumulative oestrogen exposure was centrally related to its induction and/or promotion. Thus, the effects of exogenous oestrogen on the incidence of this tumour were watched with interest. In the mid-1970s, the studies of Ziel and Finkle[3] showed conclusively that unopposed oestrogen action was associated with an excess of endometrial adenocarcinoma, a problem that led to the institution of cyclic or continuous progestogen in order to effect periodic shedding or non-proliferation of the endometrium.[4] Although largely successful in this role, the progestogens may themselves cause unacceptable adverse effects such as bloating, mastalgia and a pre-menstrual-like syndrome as well as the very bleeding whose cessation at menopause is welcomed by the great majority of women.

The breast cancer issue has been clarified in recent years with the publication of a large re-analysis of relevant studies which indicates that the risk attributable to HRT is small but undoubtedly present.[5] Many women aver that they will only accept HRT if it is accompanied by amenorrhoea and a risk of breast cancer which is, at worst, neutral. There is a further element to the rejection of HRT by a sector of the female population. Oestrogen may be the cause of an increase in libido and a woman's personal circumstances may lead to such an increase being unwelcome. Further, many women regard the cyclic changes induced by oestrogen, breast and uterus as being tantamount to the cyclic preparation for pregnancy inherent in the human menstrual cycle. Germaine Greer and others have argued that the physiological infertility and hormonal quietude of the postmenopause should not be disturbed by the resurrection of a spurious reproductive cycle.[8]

Mechanisms of action

This has been covered in detail elsewhere but it is important to restate that in the breast and endometrium the engagement of receptor by ligand requires an operational AF-2 domain of the ER for gene transcription. The function of this domain is inhibited by raloxifene, which splints Helix 12 of the ER thereby preventing its rotation and denying access by co-activators to the reconformed complex.[6] The occupation of the hydrophobic ligand-binding pocket by raloxifene not only disables the receptor but prevents its exportation to the cytoplasm for recycling, thus denying access of unliganded receptors to oestradiol. Raloxifene therefore produces a competitive blockade of ER at sites where AF-2 activity is obligatory. Conversely, the AF–1 site, which is constitutive and ligand independent, continues to function in the presence of raloxifene and permits the raloxifene–ER complex to engage the oestrogen response elements and proceed to activation of RNA polymerase II and gene transcription.

Sites of raloxifene action: uterus

Raloxifene engages the ERs that are found in the stratum basalis of the endometrium, the layer retained after menstrual shedding. The hallmark of oestrogen action is a rapid proliferation of the cells of this stratum together with the development of uncoiled endometrial glands. Stromal eosinophilia is also seen at this proliferative or pre-ovulatory stage of the female reproductive cycle. The endometrium rapidly attains a height of c. 6–10 mm by midcycle, at which stage it is primed for secretory transformation by luteal progesterone.[7] Hence, examination of the uterine safety of any putative SERM will require the gross and microscopic demonstration of endometrial and stromal inactivity with no significant increase in endometrial depth, no stromal eosinophilia and, where measurable, no significant increase in uterine dimensions and weight.

Uterine safety

The evidence of raloxifene's ability to impede oestrogen-induced endometrial proliferation goes back 16 years to the original observations of Black et al in the immature rat.[8] It was realised early that raloxifene appeared to act as a relatively pure antagonist on the endometrial ER and, unlike tamoxifen, did not appear to carry even partial agonist activity. It was further noted that raloxifene's competitive oestrogen blockade was dose-dependent, highly potent at an estimated dosage of c. 1 mg/kg and blocked the proliferative effects of tamoxifen on the mature rat endometrium.[9] At the gene-product level raloxifene has been shown to inhibit both C-*fos* expression[10] and glycogen synthesis[11] and to increase complement C production.[12]

The animal data have been well reviewed by Bryant et al[9] and indicate that although a small increase in uterine weight was observed[13] this is explained by water retention manifesting as uterine stromal oedema. In this animal model, raloxifene, in doses ranging 100-fold from 0.01 to 1.0 mg/kg, failed to produce any significant effect on stromal eosinophilia or on endometrial thickness. Indeed, raloxifene has been shown to restrain oestradiol-induced endometrial proliferation[8] and even to prevent the progression of tamoxifen-induced endometrial carcinoma in athymic mice.[14]

In women, Boss et al[15] examined the effect of 200 or 600 mg/day raloxifene and conjugated equine oestrogens on the endometrium in postmenopausal women in an 8-week placebo-controlled study. Biopsies at entry and at conclusion scored the specimens histologically on endometrial, glandular and stromal oestrogenic effects. Of the oestrogen-treated women ($n = 47$), 77% exhibited significant effects whereas in placebo-treated controls ($n = 53$) only 15% showed such changes. In the raloxifene-treated groups receiving 200 mg ($n = 54$) and 600 mg ($n = 54$), no patient exhibited marked or even moderate oestrogenic features.

In a large prospective, placebo-controlled trial, Delmas et al[16] examined, inter alia, the effects of raloxifene on double-layer endometrial thickness measured by transvaginal ultrasonography. Baseline thickness was 1.9–2.0 mm and at no time over the 2 years of the study did this value show significant change in any of the three treatment groups who received 30 mg, 60 mg and 150 mg raloxifene/day.

Raloxifene has been given to healthy premenopausal women with normal menstrual cycles in a two-part study reported by Baker et al.[17] In part I, raloxifene (400 mg/day) was given for 5 days in the follicular or luteal phases of the cycle, while in part II the agent was given for 28 days from day 3. Raloxifene did not inhibit ovulation or cycle length. Endometrial depth was measured by transvaginal ultrasonography. Endometrial biopsies obtained by the Pipelle technique were scored blindly for gland number, glandular mitotic rate and stromal mitotic rate. An assessment of the histological maturity versus the cycle day was also made.

Endometrial depth decreased non-significantly in volunteers receiving raloxifene. Histologically, the number of endometrial glands or mitoses did not change in the proliferative phase of the cycle. In the luteal phase, a 2-day dysynchrony developed in the raloxifene-treated group with the maturation lagging behind the cycle day. Overall, the authors concluded that in the presence of normal premenopausal plasma oestradiol raloxifene exerts endometrial effects that are subtle, and are not of pathological importance. A further 1-year randomized, controlled trial in postmenopausal women by Lufkin et al[18] again revealed no difference in endometrial depth between volunteers receiving 60 or 120 mg/day raloxifene and placebo-treated controls.

In summary, raloxifene appears to be highly oestrogen-antagonistic in the postmenopausal endometrium in conditions of low ambient plasma oestradiol. There is no evidence of endometrial or stromal oestrogen agonism and no dose or time-dependent effects have been observed. Confirmation is required, from the large prospective trials still underway, of the suggestion that the incidence of endometrial cancer is lower in raloxifene-treated women than in placebo-treated controls.

Breast safety

Raloxifene was first developed as a potential treatment for breast cancer and, though its primary licensed use has proved to be the prevention of osteoporosis and related fracture, considerable interest has been given to its trial results in respect of this most feared postmenopausal tumour. Attention has also been paid to symptomatic problems involving the breast because with conventional HRT, breast enlargement, nipple sensitivity and mastalgia are frequently reported by women, particularly in the early weeks of treatment.[2]

In vitro, raloxifene was found to inhibit the growth of the MCF-7 breast cancer cell line[9] and also to restrain the ability of such cells to pass an artificial basement membrane.[19] In the rat, raloxifene prevented DMBA-induced mammary tumours to a degree similar to that achieved by tamoxifen.[20] However, in humans, a single study in patients with metastatic cancer demonstrated no effects on tumour progression.[11] This was, however, a short-term study in a limited number of patients who were already known to be resistant to tamoxifen. In the intact mature rat, raloxifene induced a regression of mammary development[20] and in combination with 9-*cis*-retinoic acid, raloxifene prevented the development of mammary tumours.[21] Grodishar and colleagues reported the results of a Phase II study of raloxifene in 18 postmenopausal women with recurrent ER+

breast cancer.[22] They found that raloxifene 150 mg/b.d. for 6 months resulted in partial responses and disease stability in three and five patients, respectively. Two of the three partial responses were of over 18 months' duration. The authors found raloxifene to be well tolerated in this study, which, although small, produced response rates similar to those seen with licensed hormone treatments of advanced breast cancer.

In Phase III clinical trials in human volunteers, raloxifene has generally been found to cause no more breast tenderness than placebo-treated controls. Walsh[23] reported only a 4% incidence of breast tenderness in 95 women receiving 60 mg/day raloxifene for 6 months, a rate that compared favourably to a 35% incidence in a comparator group receiving conjugated equine oestrogen ($p = 0.001$). Lufkin et al, in their 1-year prospective trial, found that raloxifene did not occasion any symptoms attributable to breast stimulation[18] and in the largest controlled study reported to date, Delmas et al found a 3.3% incidence of mastalgia in the raloxifene groups ($n = 451$), which was not significantly different from the 2.0% incidence among the placebo-treated controls.[16] However encouraging the data on breast symptomatology, what really matters in terms of patient acceptability is the incidence of breast cancer. A report to the American Society of Clinical Oncology in 1998 presented 2-year interim data from the Phase III randomized, placebo-controlled trial of multiple outcome of raloxifene evaluation (MORE). Cummings et al reported that in a 28.9-month follow-up of 7704 postmenopausal women randomized 2:1 to raloxifene:placebo, 32 confirmed cases of invasive breast cancer had occurred in total.[24] These partitioned to 11 in the raloxifene group and 21 in the placebo group. The relative risk (95% CI) of breast cancer in the raloxifene-treated women was 0.26 (0.13–0.52). This result remained significant when adjusted for interim monitoring. Also in 1998, Jordan et al[25] reported to the San Antonio Breast Cancer Symposium on 58 cases of invasive and non-invasive breast cancer which had arisen in all placebo-controlled studies of raloxifene. This represented some 16 908 woman-years of raloxifene exposure and 8132 woman-years of placebo exposure. Median exposure was 33 months. The incidence of newly diagnosed breast cancer was 1.7 per 1000 woman-years on raloxifene and 3.7 per 1000 woman-years on placebo. The relative risk (95% CI) of breast cancer in raloxifene-treated patients was 0.46 (0.28–0.75). The overall reduction in incidence of ER+ tumours was some 70%, with no discernible effect on the incidence of ER– tumours and no selective prevention of invasive as opposed to non-invasive breast cancers. Three-year interim data from the MORE study have now been published.[26] Overall, the authors found a 76% reduction in the risk of breast cancer, over a median of 40 months, in raloxifene treated women compared to controls. Relative risk was 0.24 (0.13–0.44); $P < 0.001$. The results were again suggestive of a specific preventive action against ER+ tumours for which the relative risk in raloxifene treated women was 0.10 (0.04–0.24), whereas no effect was demonstrable against ER− tumours; relative risk 0.88 (0.26–3.0). The wide confidence intervals for ER− cancer reflect the low number of cases encountered. The number of patients in this cohort – not at high risk of breast cancer – that needed to be treated in order to prevent one case of breast cancer, was 126. Thus the evolving data show an encouraging trend and internal consistency.

These data allow for cautious optimism in respect of raloxifene and breast cancer. The probability of a true preventive or suppressive effect is enhanced by the observation that, as with tamoxifen, the protective effect appears to be confined to oestrogen receptor positive (ER+) tumours.[25] The fact that the incidence of breast tumours in the control group was that expected in the population studied is also encouraging, as is the failure of raloxifene to opacify the breast to mammography which should mitigate against false negative reporting. It should be noted, however, that populations with osteoporosis, such as studied by MORE, may be at a lower than average risk of breast cancer and hence the above observation should not be transposed to populations at high risk. Indeed, in the USA, a prospective study that will compare raloxifene and tamoxifen in a high-risk population is now in recruitment.

It should be cautioned that the biology of raloxifene action on the breast is far from being completely understood. Thus, the breast cancers that are failing to manifest during the above trials may be being suppressed rather than primarily prevented. It will therefore be absolutely necessary to maintain vigilance over trial patients ceasing to take raloxifene by continuing with studies of sufficient power to detect any significant deviation from the rate of breast cancer expected in that population.

Conclusions

From the data available it appears that raloxifene is truly antagonistic to the oestrogen-sensitive tissues of breast and uterus. Patients receiving the drug for its licensed indication of bone loss and fracture prevention may be reassured that there is no evidence of an increased risk of uterine or breast cancer and that, with the latter, the reverse may indeed by the case. The absence of breast symptoms and of vaginal bleeding should prove a major asset in this agent's acceptability and the degree of protection against breast cancer may yet form the basis of an application to the regulatory authorities for an extension of the licence. Any oestrogen replacement regimen must, at base, be bleed-free and breast-safe for it to commend itself to long-term continuation by women after menopause.

Over 100 years ago in Glasgow, Beatson, in what is now a classic paper in oncology, observed that oophorectomy resulted in the clinical improvement in some but not all women with advanced breast cancer.[27] With hindsight, Beatson was probably observing the positive effect of acute oestrogen and progestogen withdrawal in cases of ER+ tumours, a receptor modulation by surgical removal of ligand. Now, over a century later, the molecular jigsaw of breast cancer is, to use Fentiman's graphic phrase, still in fragments, although the advent of medical receptor modulation by SERMs may yet prove a means to join together several of the pieces.

References

1. *Raloxifene: Summary of Product Characteristics.* Medicines Control Agency: London.
2. Purdie DW, Steel SA, Howey S, Doherty SM. The technical and logistical feasibility of population densitometry using DXA and directed HRT intervention: a 2-year prospective study. *Osteoporos Int* 1996; **11**: S31–6.
3. Ziel H, Finkle W. Increased risk of endometrial carcinoma among users of conjugated estrogens. *N Engl J Med* 1975; **293**: 1167.
4. Col NF, Eckman MH, Karas RH et al. Patient-specific decisions about hormone replacement therapy in postmenopausal women. *JAMA* 1997; **14**: 1140–7.
5. Collaborative Group on Hormonal Factors in Breast Cancer. Breast cancer and hormonal contraceptives: collaborative re-analysis of individual data on 53 297 women with breast cancer and 100 239 women without breast cancer from 54 epidemiological studies. *Lancet* 1996; **347**: 1713–27.
6. Brzozowski AM, Pike ACW, Dauter Z et al. Molecular basis of agonism and antagonism in the oestrogen receptor. *Nature* 1997; **389**: 753–8.
7. Ferenczy A, Bertrand G, Gelfand MM. Proliferation kinetics of human endometrium during the normal menstrual cycle. *Am J Obstet Gynecol* 1979; **133**: 859–67.
8. Black LJ, Jones CD, Falcone JF. Antagonism of estrogen action with a new benzothiophene derived anti-estrogen. *Life Sci* 1983; **32**: 1031–6.
9. Bryant HU, Glasebrook AL, Yang NN, Sato M. A pharmacological review of raloxifene. *J Bone Miner Metab* 1996; **14**: 1–9.
10. Pellerin I, Vuillermoz C, Jouvenot M et al. Superinduction of *c-Fos* gene expression by estrogen in cultured guinea pig endometrial cells requires priming by a cycloheximide-dependent mechanism. *Endocrinology* 1992; **131**: 1094–100.
11. Buzdar AU, Marcus C, Holmes F et al. Phase II evaluation of LY156758 in metastatic breast cancer. *Oncology* 1988; **45**: 344–5.
12. Sundstrom S, Komm BS, Xu Q et al. The stimulation of uterine complement C3 gene expression by antiestrogens. *Endocrinology* 1990; **126**: 1449–56.
13. Szego C, Roberts S. Steroid action and interactions in uterine metabolism. *Recent Prog Horm Res* 1953; **8**: 419–68.
14. Gottardis MM, Richio ME. Satyaswaroop PG, Jordan VC. Effect of steroidal and nonsteroidal antiestrogens on the growth of a tamoxifen-stimulated human endometrial

carcinoma (EnCa101) in athymic mice. *Cancer Res* 1990; **50**: 3189–92.

15. Boss SM, Huster WJ, Neild JA et al. Effects of raloxifene hydrochloride on the endometrium of postmenopausal women. *Am J Obstet Gynecol* 1997; **177**: 1458–64.

16. Delmas PD, Bjarnason NH, Mitlak BH et al. Effects of raloxifene on bone mineral density, serum cholesterol concentrations and uterine endometrium in postmenopausal women. *N Engl J Med* 1997; **337**: 1641–7.

17. Baker VL, Draper M, Paul S et al. Reproductive endocrine and endometrial effects of raloxifene hydrochloride, a selective estrogen receptor modulator, in women with regular menstrual cycles. *J Clin Endocrinol Metab* 1998; **83**: 6–13.

18. Lufkin EG, Whitaker MD, Nickelsen T et al. Treatment of established postmenopausal osteoporosis with raloxifene: a randomized trial. *J Bone Miner Res* 1998; **13**: 1747–54.

19. Thompson EW, Reich R, Shima TB et al. Differential regulation of growth and invasiveness of MCF-7 breast cancer cells by antiestrogens. *Cancer Res* 1988; **48**: 6764–8.

20. Clemens JA, Bennett DR, Black LJ, Jones CD. Effects of a new anti-estrogen, keoxifene LY156758 on growth of carcinogen-induced mammary tumours and on LH and prolactin levels. *Life Sci* 1983; **32**: 2869–75.

21. Anzano MA, Peer CW, Smith JM et al. Chemoprevention of mammary carcinogenesis in the rat: combined use of raloxifene and 9-cis-retinoic acid. *J Natl Cancer Inst* 1996; **88**: 123–5.

22. Grodishar WJ. The effect of raloxifene on the risk of breast cancer in post menopausal women. *20th American San Antonio Breast Cancer Symposium*, San Antonio, Texas, December 1997.

23. Walsh BW, Kuller LH, Wild RA et al. Effects of raloxifene on serum lipids and coagulation factors in healthy postmenopausal women. *JAMA* 1998; **279**: 1445–51.

24. Cummings SR, Norton L, Eckert S et al. Raloxifene reduces the risk of breast cancer and may decrease the risk of endometrial cancer in post-menopausal women. Two-year findings from the multiple outcomes of raloxifene evaluation (MORE) trial. *Proceedings of the American Society of Clinical Oncology 34th annual meeting*, May 1998. WB Saunders/Mack Printing Group: Philadelphia, 1998: 2a, Abstract 3.

25. Jordan VC, Glusman JE, Eckert S et al. Raloxifene reduces incident primary breast cancers: integrated data from multicenter, double-blind, placebo-controlled, randomized trials in postmenopausal women. *20th American San Antonio Breast Cancer Symposium*, San Antonio, Texas, December 1997: Abstract 2.

26. Cummings SR, Eckert S, Krueger KA et al. The effect of raloxifene on risk of breast cancer in postmenopausal women: results from the MORE randomized trial. *JAMA* 1999; **281**: 2189–97.

27. Beatson GT. On the treatment of inoperable cases of carcinoma of the mamma: suggestions for a new method of treatment with illustrative cases. *Lancet* 1896; **ii**: 162–7.

10

SERMs: other aspects of the safety profile

Donato Agnusdei, Nicoletta Iori

Based on the data available today, SERMs, particularly raloxifene, present a very good clinical safety profile. The major side effect is the increased risk of venous thromboembolism with a magnitude comparable to tamoxifen and HRT.

Introduction

Previous chapters have described the safety profile of selective oestrogen receptor modulators (SERMs) in the reproductive system. This chapter will report the other safety aspects of the clinically available SERMs, namely tamoxifen and raloxifene Knowledge about the clinical safety of SERMs comes from experience with the triphenylethylene SERM tamoxifen, which is widely used for treatment of breast cancer, as well as from extensive, ongoing clinical trials with raloxifene, a benzothiophene SERM currently available for clinical use to prevent osteoporosis in postmenopausal women.

Clinical safety

Tamoxifen is the most extensively studied SERM, with literally millions of patient-years exposure since its initial use to treat advanced breast cancer in the early 1970s. Since then, tamoxifen has become the treatment of choice, not only for advanced disease, but also for early breast cancer, where it has been extensively investigated and used in clinical practice for nearly 20 years. However, there is substantially less clinical experience with tamoxifen in healthy postmenopausal women, and much of what we know about tamoxifen in healthy women has come from the recently published trials performed in the USA and Europe. [1–3] In these trials, two non-serious adverse events, hot flushes and vaginal discharge, were reported significantly more frequently by women receiving tamoxifen compared with placebo. Tamoxifen increased both the frequency and severity of hot flushes relative to placebo. These findings are consistent with data from other large adjuvant trials of tamoxifen in postmenopausal breast cancer patients.[4,5]

Treatment with tamoxifen is also associated with an increased risk of cataracts and cataract surgery. Several trials have linked tamoxifen to retinal crystal formation after prolonged use, but the clinical impact of this is uncertain, since the crystals do not seem to interfere with vision.[1,3] Tamoxifen has also been associated with liver enzyme elevations but they are usually mild and asymptomatic; severe liver abnormalities have been reported only rarely. Although tamoxifen causes liver cancer in rats, it does not appear to do the same in humans.[5] Furthermore, other side effects, such as nausea, vomiting, and gastric discomfort have been reported among women with metastatic breast cancer treated with tamoxifen. It is difficult to determine whether some of these so-called reactions are related to tamoxifen or a consequence of the disease state.

The other SERM with extensive clinical trial experience in postmenopausal women is raloxifene. Raloxifene was synthesized in 1979 and was first called keoxifene. Since then, about 14 000 postmenopausal women have participated in clinical trials, nearly 11 000 of whom have participated in placebo-controlled trials with a median duration of 40 months. Most of these trials were designed to test the safety and efficacy of raloxifene in the prevention and treatment of osteoporosis, and they also provide the extensive safety database for raloxifene. A significantly greater number of women have been recently exposed to marketed raloxifene, with safety data thus far consistent with clinical trial findings. The two non-serious side effects which have been linked to raloxifene therapy in some women are hot flushes and leg cramps.

Treatment of vasodilatation ('hot flushes') is a major reason for taking hormone replacement therapy (HRT) in the early postmenopausal period. Based on clinical trial data, raloxifene is not suitable for acute use in perimenopausal or early postmenopausal women who have pre-existing vasomotor instability. It may cause or worsen this symptom in women who are asymptomatic or have mild pre-existing symptoms.[6] Early evidence for this comes from a Phase II trial where high-dose raloxifene 600 mg/day caused a statistically significantly greater frequency of hot flushes compared with placebo after 8 weeks.[7] These data were confirmed in a recent analysis from five large, randomized, placebo-controlled osteoporosis prevention trials involving 1165 healthy, postmenopausal women (mean age, 54 years).[8] After a median of 30 months' exposure to raloxifene, the number of women reporting hot flushes (25%) in the 60-mg dose of raloxifene was significantly higher than the placebo group (18%). However, the rate of study discontinuations due to hot flushes was comparable between the raloxifene 60 mg and placebo groups (~2% per group).[9] Moreover, in the same analysis, the occurrence of a related vasomotor symptom, sweating (which includes night sweats), was not statistically different for the raloxifene- or placebo-treated subjects.[8]

Hot flushes were also reported in the larger Multiple Outcomes Raloxifene Evaluation (MORE) trial, although the cumulative incidence of women with at least one hot flush episode is much lower in MORE compared with the osteoporosis prevention studies. This is because hot flushes decrease with age, and the women enrolled in MORE were about 12 years older on average (mean age, 66 years) than the early healthy postmenopausal women enrolled in osteoporosis prevention trials. In MORE, 6.4% of placebo patients and 9.7% of raloxifene 60-mg patients reported hot flushes; less than 1% reported their worst episode as severe.[10] In comparison, 2% of prevention patients reported their worst hot flush episode as severe; this incidence is lower than the incidence observed in patients treated with tamoxifen.[5]

The other non-serious side effect linked with raloxifene administration is idiopathic leg cramps; these were reported by about 6% of women treated with raloxifene for 2 years compared with about 2% receiving a placebo in placebo-controlled osteoporosis prevention trials. All were reported as mild or moderate.[8] The incidence of leg cramps was comparable between the raloxifene and HRT groups in the HRT-controlled database. No statistical difference was observed between patients treated with raloxifene and unopposed oestrogen.[8] It should be noted that leg cramps is a side effect frequently reported in postmenopausal women treated long-term with HRT.[11] In patients receiving raloxifene this symptom was not associated with body fluid retention or any alteration in the electrolyte and/or mineral metabolism.

Venous Thromboembolic Events (VTE)

Venous thromboembolism (VTE) is a rare but serious group of disorders in the general population. The most common manifestation is deep venous thrombosis (DVT); less common is pulmonary embolus. An estimated one person per 1000 at age 60 is affected by VTE annually, and this risk doubles approximately every 10 years.[12] Oestrogens have been associated with increased VTE risk. These risks have been more highly attributed to the high-dose oestrogens in oral contraceptive pills; second and third generation contraceptive pills were recently stated to have an even higher risk of VTE.[13] Four recent epidemiological studies highlighted the increased risk, two- to fourfold, of DVT or pulmonary emboli associated with HRT. It is important to note that the databases upon which these studies are based included relatively few women over age 65.[14–17]

Figure 10.1 summarizes the VTE results from two recent observational studies of hormone replacement therapy,[16,17] one prospective clinical trial of continuous-combined oestrogen-progestin hormone replacement therapy in women with heart disease (HERS),[18] one prospective clinical trial of tamoxifen known as P-1,[1] and the prospective placebo-controlled clinical trial experience with raloxifene. In these studies, the VTE relative risks for HRT and SERM users compared to non-users are all between 2 and 4. The incidence rate for all reported cases is available only from the prospective clinical trials, since the observational studies limited their analyses to idiopathic cases only. In the MORE study, postmenopausal women with osteoporosis treated for three years with raloxifene, had a relative risk of VTE of 3.1 (95% CI 1.5–6.2).[10] The incidence rates for the tamoxifen and raloxifene trials are similar. The higher incidence in the HERS study reflects the higher baseline trial risk of women in this study, because the study cohort was composed exclusively of women with prior heart disease. Therefore, oestrogens and drugs with oestrogen actions increase the risk of venous thromboembolism to a similar degree, although the mechanism is not known.

Effects of SERMs on neuropsychomotor and cognitive function

Preclinical studies suggest that oestrogens may affect central nervous system function, enhancing cholinergic and serotoninergic mechanisms in the rat brain and modulating the growth and maintenance of neuronal cells in vitro.[19] Nevertheless, the effect of oestrogen on cognitive function in humans remains a matter of debate. In postmenopausal women, modest improvement in certain aspects of

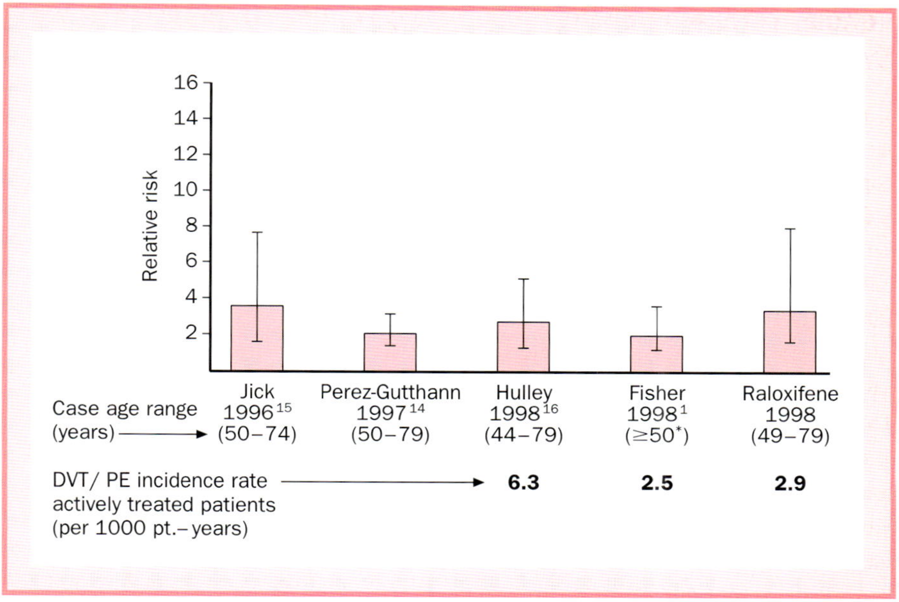

Figure 10.1
Relative risk for deep venous thrombosis (DVT), and pulmonary emboli (PE) in women treated with HRT, tamoxifen and raloxifene. Results from five prospective randomised, placebo-controlled trials.
** Analysis restricted to age group.*

cognitive function, particularly in verbal memory, have been demonstrated after oestrogen administration. Several epidemiological studies suggest that oestrogen replacement therapy may delay the onset of Alzheimer's disease,[20] although in other studies no effect was observed.[21] Thus, confirmation of any positive effect on cognition, as well as clarification of its magnitude and clinical significance, must await completion of large scale, randomized, placebo-controlled, prospective trials.[21]

Several cognitive evaluation tools have been used to investigate whether raloxifene therapy has a beneficial effect on cognitive function. Overall, there is no evidence of a deleterious effect of raloxifene therapy on cognitive function. This is consistent with information recently published from a Phase II trial.[22] This observation, together with the preclinical observations that raloxifene has oestrogen agonist properties in the hippocampus,[23] suggest that raloxifene may act as an oestrogen-receptor agonist on cognitive function. These findings have been recently confirmed in a study showing that raloxifene is an oestrogen agonist in inducing the outgrowth of neurites in nerve-growth-factor-treated PC 12 cells. These cells express both oestrogen receptor α and β.[24]

Data from the MORE study showed that the incidence of cognitive decline from baseline over 3 years is low in this population. Prospective clinical data are also not yet available for oestrogens, although some believe that oestrogens will eventually demonstrate a beneficial effect on cognitive function.[20,21]

In a recent analysis performed in several placebo controlled studies using raloxifene, there was no evidence that raloxifene was associated with adverse events in the central nervous system. No differences among treatment groups have been found for depressive symptoms, emotional lability, insomnia, anxiety, dizziness, malaise and amnesia.[8]

In patients with established postmenopausal osteoporosis enrolled in MORE, neuropsychomotor testing revealed no consistent beneficial or deleterious effects of raloxifene on key endpoints such as static balance, gait, and falls. The results of these tests are consistent with adverse event data related to the frequency of falls and accidents. Maintenance of neuropsychomotor integrity is important because falls are the leading cause of peripheral fractures in postmenopausal women, with 1 fall in 100 resulting in a fracture.[25–27]

Effects of raloxifene on quality of life

The most important observation from quality of life evaluations in raloxifene trials is that both prevalent and incident vertebral fractures have a deleterious effect on quality of life. These data corroborate published observations where the overall impact of incident osteoporotic vertebral fractures is comparable to that from disability in arthritis or diabetes mellitus.[28] In the MORE trial, no overall beneficial or deleterious effect was seen in the subset of patients evaluated with disease-specific instruments such as OPAQ (Osteoporosis Assessment Questionnaire) and QualEFFO (European Foundation for Osteoporosis Quality-of-life Questionnaire).[29] Overall, chronic raloxifene therapy is well-tolerated.

Raloxifene: drug interactions

Raloxifene dose not compete with protein binding sites for medicines such as tamoxifen, phenytoin, and warfarin. As expected, single doses of warfarin do not alter steady-state plasma raloxifene concentrations, but raloxifene did reduce by 10% the effect of a large single dose (20 mg) of warfarin on prothrombin time through a pharmacodynamic mechanism. However, in clinical practice, raloxifene would either be added to chronic warfarin use, or routinely used doses of warfarin (eg, 5.0 mg daily) would be added to chronic raloxifene use. Given this pharmacodynamic interaction, it is recommended to carefully monitor prothrombin times whenever raloxifene is given concurrently with warfarin or other coumarin derivatives.

In classical pharmacokinetic analyses for drug-drug interactions, there were no clinically significant interactions observed between raloxifene and the following: digoxin, calcium carbonate, aluminium- and magnesium-hydroxide-containing antacids, and ampicillin. Not surprisingly, cholestyramine reduces the absorption and enterohepatic cycling of raloxifene, so these two medicines should not be used concomitantly.

The influence of concomitant medication on raloxifene plasma concentrations was evaluated in the osteoporosis prevention trials.[6] Frequently co-administered drugs included: acetaminophen, non-steroidal anti-inflammatory drugs (such as aspirin, ibuprofen, and naproxen), oral antibiotics, H_1 antagonists, H_2 antagonists, and benzodiazepines. No clinically relevant effects of the co-administration of the agents on raloxifene disposition were identified. Based on analyses from these studies, raloxifene may be administered without regard to food intake, age, body weight, cigarette smoking, ethnic origin, alcohol use, routinely used medications, and decreased renal function associated with ageing.

Conclusion

Based on currently available data, the clinical safety profile of SERMs, particularly raloxifene, seems to be excellent. SERMs hold great promise for maintaining the long-term health of postmenopausal women.

References

1. Fisher B, Costantino JP, Wickerham DL et al. Tamoxifen for prevention of breast cancer: report from the National Surgical Adjuvant Breast and Bowel Project P-1 study. *J Natl Cancer Inst* 1998; **90**: 1371–88.
2. Powles T, Eeles, R, Ashley S et al. Interim analysis of the incidence of breast cancer in the Royal Marsden Hospital tamoxifen randomised chemoprevention trial. *Lancet* 1998; **352**: 98–101.
3. Veronesi U, Maisonneuve P, Costa A et al. Prevention of breast cancer with tamoxifen: preliminary findings from the Italian randomised trial among hysterectomised women. *Lancet* 1998; **352**: 93–7.
4. Osborne CK: Tamoxifen in the treatment of breast cancer. *N Engl J Med* 1998; **339**: 1609–18.
5. Fisher B, Costantino JP, Redmond CK et al. Endometrial cancer in tamoxifen-treated breast cancer patients: findings from the National Surgical Adjuvant Breast and Bowel Project (NSABP) B-14. *J Natl Cancer Inst* 1994; **86**: 527–37.
6. Delmas PD, Bjarnason NH, Mitlak B et al. Effects of raloxifene on bone mineral density, serum cholesterol concentrations, and uterine endometrium in postmenopausal women. *N Engl J Med* 1997; **337**: 1641–7.

7. Hol T, Cox MB, Bryant HU et al. Selective estrogen receptor modulators and postmenopausal women's health. *J Women's Health* 1997; **6**: 523–31.

8. Davies GC, Lu WJ, Huster Y et al. Adverse events reported by postmenopausal women in controlled trials with raloxifene. *Obstet Gynecol* 1999; **93**: 558–65.

9. Lu Y, Cohen FJ, Lakshmanan M. Characterization of hot flashes during raloxifenetherapy: analyses of adverse event reports from an integrated placebo-controlled clinical trial database. *Menopause* 1998; **95**: Abstract 98.

10. Cummings SR, Eckert S, Krueger K et al. The effect of raloxifene on risk of breast cancer in postmenopausal women. *JAMA* 1999; **281**: 2189–97.

11. Campbell S, Whitehead M. Oestrogen therapy and the menopausal syndrome. *Clin Obstet Gynaecol* 1997; 4(**1**): 31–47.

12. Kniffin WD Jr, Baron JA, Barrett J et al. The epidemiology of diagnosed pulmonary embolism and deep venous thrombosis in the elderly. *Arch Intern Med* 1994; **154**: 861–6.

13. Vandenbroucke JP, Koster T, Briet E et al. Increased risk of venous thrombosis in oral-contraceptive users who are carriers of factor V Leiden mutation. *Lancet* 1996; **344**: 1453–7.

14. Daly E, Vessey MP, Hawkins MM et al. Risk of venous thromboembolism in users of hormone replacement therapy. *Lancet* 1996; **348**: 977–80.

15. Grodstein F, Stampfer MJ, Goldhaber SZ et al. Prospective study of exogeneous hormones and risk of pulmonary embolism in women. *Lancet* 1996; **348**: 983–7.

16. Gutthann SP, Rodriguez LAG, Castellsague J et al. Hormone replacement therapy and risk of venous thromboembolism: population based case control study. *Br Med J* 1997; **314**: 796–800.

17. Jick H, Derby LE, Myers MW et al. Risk of hospital admission for idiopathic venous thromboembolism among users of postmenopausal oestrogens. *Lancet* 1996; **348**: 981–3.

18. Hulley SB, Grady D, Bush TL et al. Randomised trial of estrogen plus progestin for secondary prevention of coronary heart disease in postmenopausal women. *JAMA* 1998; **280**: 605–13.

19. Schneider LS, Finch CE. Can estrogens prevent neurodegeneration? *Drugs and Aging* 1997; **11**: 87–5.

20. Paganini-Hill A, Henderson VW. Estrogen replacement therapy and risk of Alzheimer disease. *Arch Intern Med* 1996; **156**: 2213–17.

21. Yaffe C, Sawaya G, Lieberburg I et al. Estrogen therapy in postmenopausal women. Effects on cognitive function and dementia. *JAMA* 1998; **279**: 688–95.

22. Nickelsen T, Lufkin EG, Riggs BL et al. Raloxifene hydrochloride, a selective estrogen receptor modulator: safety assessment of effects on cognitive function and mood in postmenopausal women. *Psychoneuroendocrinology* 1999; **24**: 115–28.

23. Lorenzo A, Diaz H, Carrer HF et al. Amygdala neurons in vitro: neurite growth and effects of estradiol. *J Neurosci Res* 1992; **33**: 418–35.

24. Nilsen J, Mor G, Naftolin F. Raloxifene induces neurite outgrowth in estrogen receptor positive PC12 cells. *Menopause* 1998; **5**: 211–16.

25. Cumming SR, Nevitt MC. Falls (Editorial). *N Engl J Med* 1994; **331(13)**: 872–3.

26. Dargent-Molina P, Favier F, Grandjean H et al. Hausherr E, Meunier PJ, Breart G. Fall-related factors and risk of hip fracture: the EPIDOS prospective study. *Lancet* 1996: **348**: 145–9.

27. Graafmans WC, Ooms ME, Hofstee HMA et al. Falls in the elderly: a prospective study of risk factors and risk profiles. *Am J Epidemiol* 1996; **143(11)**: 1129–36.

28. Nevitt MC, Ettinger B, Black DM et al. The association of radiographically detected vertebral fractures with back pain and function: a prospective study. *Ann Intern Med* 1998; **128**: 793–800.

29. Lips P, Cooper C, Agnusdei D. Quality of life in patients with vertebral fractures: validation of the quality of life questionnaire of the European Foundation for Osteoporosis (QUALEFFO). *Osteoporosis Int* 1999; **10**: 150–1.

11

The role of SERMS in clinical practice

Juliet Compston

SERMs provide a new option for the management of postmenopausal osteoporosis and raloxifene has recently been licenced for this indication. The choice of agent depends on a number of factors including anti-fracture efficacy, site-specificity, adverse effects and extraskeletal risks and benefits. The emerging pharmacological profile of raloxifene indicates a good risk/benefit ratio and emphasises the potential for SERMs to protect against many of the major diseases of the postmenopause.

Introduction

The ability of selective oestrogen receptor modulators (SERMs) to exhibit tissue specificity and increasing insights into how such effects may be achieved have created intense interest in the potential for such compounds to prevent and treat a wide variety of diseases related to oestrogen status. Such conditions include osteoporosis, breast cancer, coronary heart disease and possibly also cerebrovascular disease and dementia: although at present the therapeutic use of SERMs is targeted at postmenopausal women, these compounds also have considerable potential application in premenopausal women and men. The widespread distribution of oestrogen receptors and the diversity of actions of the hormone present intriguing opportunities for the manipulation of oestrogen signalling pathways and hence optimization of the pharmacological profile of receptor modulators. At present, however, the clinical use of SERMs is limited to breast cancer and osteoporosis; for the latter condition only one product, namely raloxifene, is licensed. This chapter reviews the role of raloxifene in the prevention of osteoporotic fractures in the context of other currently available interventions and considers possible clinical applications of SERMs in the future.

Prevention of osteoporotic fractures: current options

General considerations

There have been significant advances in the management of osteoporosis in recent years and a number of agents are now licensed for its prevention and treatment (***Table 11.1***). The level of evidence for efficacy of these interventions varies considerably; for example, nearly all the fracture data on hormone replacement therapy (HRT) are based on observational studies in which beneficial effects are likely to be overestimated, and evidence from adequately powered randomized controlled trials with fracture as the primary endpoint exists only for alendronate, raloxifene and combined vitamin D and calcium.

Although management of osteoporosis has traditionally been separated into prevention and treatment, this distinction is not useful in clinical practice and the endpoint of intervention in all patients is the prevention of osteoporotic fracture, whether or not previous fractures have occurred. Nearly all the agents currently licensed for osteoporosis act predominantly by suppressing bone resorption; characteristically their use is associated with a small and transient increase in bone mineral density as a result of in-filling of the remodelling space; in contrast, anabolic agents such as sodium fluoride and parathyroid hormone produce larger, sustained increases in bone mineral density (***Figure 11.1***).[1] However, there is evidence from several treatment studies that the magnitude of reduction in fracture achieved with antiresorptive drugs is considerably greater than can be explained on the basis of changes in bone mineral density alone[2] and effects on cancellous bone structure and, for some drugs, on muscle strength and postural stability, may also contribute to protection against fracture. Conversely, large increases in bone mineral density may be associated with increased fracture risk, as demonstrated in some studies with sodium fluoride.[3]

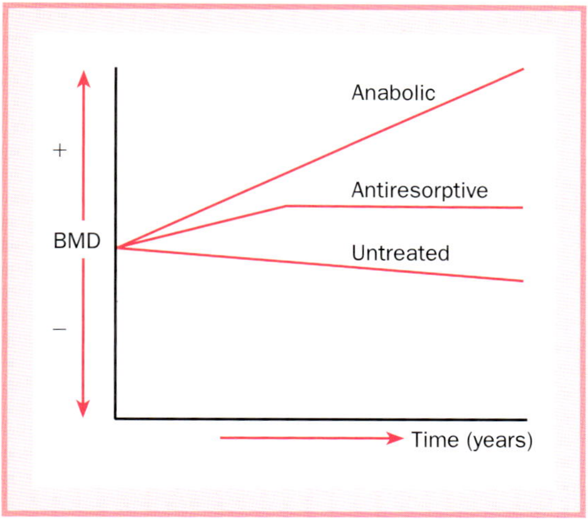

Figure 11.1
Effects on bone mass of antiresorptive and anabolic agents. (Reprinted with permission from ref. 1.)

Hormone replacement therapy

The role of oestrogen deficiency in the pathogenesis of postmenopausal osteoporosis is well established. Oral, transdermal and parenteral formulations of oestrogen, with or without a progestogen, prevent menopausal bone loss and observational studies have documented a reduction of fracture risk at the hip, wrist and spine.[4–8] The optimal timing and duration of treatment are uncertain but there is growing evidence that skeletal benefits are maintained only with continued treatment; thus, attenuation of beneficial effects on both bone mass and fracture rate after cessation of therapy has been reported,[9,10] and the risk of hip fracture 5 years or more after withdrawal of treatment appears to revert to that of untreated women. The minimum duration of therapy required to achieve a reduction in fracture risk also remains to be established, although some observational data indicate that at least 5 years may be necessary. The beneficial skeletal effects of HRT, at least in terms of preservation of bone mineral density, are not confined to perimenopausal women but are also seen in more elderly women.[11] However, side effects are generally more troublesome in the elderly and compliance is correspondingly lower.

Short-term side effects of HRT include breast tenderness and withdrawal bleeding.

Table 11.1
Current options for the prevention of osteoporotic fractures in postmenopausal women.

Accepted antifracture efficacy at vertebral and non-vertebral sites:
hormone replacement therapy
bisphosphonates
Accepted antifracture efficacy in the spine:
raloxifene
Accepted antifracture efficacy at non-vertebral sites:
calcium and vitamin D
Possible antifracture efficacy in the spine:
calcitriol
calcitonin
calcium
sodium fluoride
Possible antifracture efficacy in the hip:
vitamin D

The latter is a major cause of non-compliance and although continuous combined 'no-bleed' formulations are now available, up to 30% of women experience some vaginal bleeding during the first few months of use of these preparations. In the context of osteoporosis, for which indefinite treatment is required to maintain maximal protection against fracture, the extraskeletal risks and benefits are particularly relevant. Long-term HRT is associated with an increase in the risk of breast cancer,[12,13] the magnitude of which is in the order of 30% and highly significant in terms of absolute risk for a disease that affects one in 12 of all postmenopausal women. There is also an increase in the risk of venous thromboembolic events[14–17] and endometrial cancer risk may also be increased in long-term users of combined HRT.[18]

In contrast with these adverse effects, HRT may have important extraskeletal benefits. Observational data indicate a significant reduction in coronary heart disease[19] in oestrogen users; this remains to be confirmed in prospective studies, but is potentially the most important effect overall of HRT in view of the high prevalence and significant morbidity and mortality attributable to this condition in postmenopausal women. However, there is evidence from a recent study that combined HRT may not be effective in the secondary prevention of coronary heart disease in postmenopausal women.[20] Observational studies indicate that use of HRT may be associated with improved cognitive function and a reduction in the risk of Alzheimer's disease.[21] Finally, HRT may be associated with a reduced risk of cancer of the colon.[22]

Bisphosphonates

Bisphosphonates are synthetic analogues of inorganic pyrophosphate. Two of these compounds are currently licensed for use in osteoporosis, namely etidronate and alendronate; the former is administered cyclically and intermittently, as a 400 mg/day dose for 2 weeks followed by calcium only for 76 days, whereas alendronate is given as a single daily dose of 10 mg. Calcium is not included in the formulation of alendronate but is recommended in patients with a low dietary intake.

Both these bisphosphonates prevent bone loss in the spine and hip, both in healthy perimenopausal women and in women with postmenopausal osteoporosis.[23–26] There is also, at least in the case of alendronate, a sustained although small increase in bone mineral density, probably attributable to hypermineralization of bone, which occurs as a consequence of reduced bone turnover.[27] Clinical trials with cyclical etidronate were not adequately powered to demonstrate significant reductions in fracture rate, although a favourable trend was seen for vertebral fractures after 3 years of treatment,[28,29] and observational data from the General Practice Research Database also support protective effects against hip and other non-vertebral fractures.[30] In the case of alendronate, a reduction of approximately 50% in vertebral, hip and wrist fracture rates has been shown in women with postmenopausal osteoporosis.[31] Although no direct comparison can be made of the antifracture efficacy of etidronate and alendronate, the similarity in changes in bone mineral density with the two agents suggests that they are likely to be comparable in this respect. Both agents have also been shown to be effective in the primary prevention of glucocorticoid-induced bone loss, with a trend towards reduction in vertebral fracture rate.[32,33]

Bisphosphonates are generally well tolerated although gastrointestinal side effects may occur, particularly with aminobisphosphonates and a small number of cases of erosive oesophagitis have been reported in patients taking alendronate.[34] This drug is therefore contraindicated in women with a history of oesophageal disease and should be used with caution in those with dyspepsia.

The optimum duration of bisphosphonate therapy is unknown. At present, treatment with cyclical etidronate or alendronate is often given for a period of 3–5 years; preliminary data suggest that bone loss resumes soon after discontinuation of treatment, although further studies are required in this area.[35]

Calcitonin

Calcitonin inhibits bone resorption by direct actions on the osteoclast. Whether given parenterally or intranasally, it prevents spinal bone loss in postmenopausal women although there is less benefit at other sites such as the proximal femur and radius.[36] In a 3-year randomized controlled study of intranasal calcitonin in women with postmenopausal osteoporosis, a significant reduction in vertebral fracture was seen in women treated with 200 IU daily, but not in those receiving 100 or 400 IU daily.[37] No significant treatment benefits in spinal bone mineral density were observed in any of the treatment groups and, particularly in view of the very high drop-out rate in this study (nearly 50%), the antifracture efficacy of calcitonin cannot be regarded as definitively established.

Adverse effects with intranasal calcitonin are rare. Parenteral calcitonin may be associated with nausea and flushing shortly after injection and diarrhoea and vomiting occasionally occur. These symptoms are usually transient but may persist for some hours.

Vitamin D

There is increasing evidence that vitamin D supplementation in the elderly protects against non-vertebral fractures.[38] In a randomized controlled trial of vitamin D and calcium in a daily dose of 800 IU and 1.2 g, respectively, in elderly women living in sheltered accommodation, a significant reduction in hip and other non-vertebral fractures was observed after 12–18 months of treatment.[39] More recently, significant protection against non-vertebral fractures was reported in community-dwelling elderly men and women after treatment with 700 IU of vitamin D daily and 500 mg/day of calcium.[40] The relative contributions of calcium and vitamin D to the observed benefits cannot be deduced from these studies; vitamin D without calcium supplements has been reported in some but not all studies to reduce the non-vertebral fracture rate in the elderly,[41,42] but the important question of whether vitamin D alone reduces hip fracture remains unanswered at present.

Vitamin D metabolites and analogues

A reduction in vertebral fracture rate has been reported in some studies for calcitriol (1,25-dihydroxyvitamin D, the active metabolite of vitamin D) and alfacalcidol (1α-hydroxyvitamin D_3) an analogue of calcitriol;[43,44] however, this finding has not been universal.[45] Both agents preserve bone mineral density in the hip, spine and total body, but as yet their effects on non-vertebral fracture rate are unknown. The dosages of calcitriol and alfacalcidol for use in osteoporosis are generally between 0.5 and 1.0 μg daily. Hypercalcaemia and hypercalciuria may occur and serum calcium levels should be monitored regularly.

Calcium

Calcium supplementation has beneficial effects on bone mass in children and adults. These have been shown most consistently at appendicular skeletal sites and are less evident in lumbar spinal bone, where the effects may be transient.[46,47] In the years during and immediately after the menopause, when oestrogen deficiency predominates, the effects of calcium are less marked. Several small studies have reported a beneficial effect of calcium supplementation on vertebral fracture rate, but evidence from adequately powered studies is lacking[48] and calcium should be regarded as an adjunct to treatment rather than a definitive therapy.

Sodium fluoride

Sodium fluoride increases bone formation via stimulation of osteoblasts. Its use in the treatment of postmenopausal osteoporosis is controversial;[3] increases in spinal bone mineral density of around 5% per year have not been associated with a reduction in vertebral fracture in all studies[49,50] and there are concerns that impaired quality of newly formed bone and neutral or even negative effects at sites where cortical bone predominates may increase the risk of non-vertebral fractures. Sodium fluoride is licensed for treatment of postmenopausal osteoporosis in some European countries, but not in the UK or USA.

The role of raloxifene in the prevention of osteoporotic fractures

Issues relevant to the positioning of interventions for osteoporosis include antifracture efficacy, site-specificity, cost, adverse effects and, particularly in the case of HRT and SERMs, potential extraskeletal risks and benefits. In addition, the timing of the onset and offset of skeletal effects may influence the choice of treatment. Whilst information on some of these aspects is available, for others there is insufficient knowledge to permit meaningful comparisons between agents. In many situations, therefore, the preferences and prejudices of individual patients (and their doctors) will influence management decisions.

Antifracture efficacy

No direct comparison of the antifracture efficacy of current therapeutic options is possible: first, because of the different levels of evidence available and, secondly, because of differences between the populations studied in clinical trials, with respect to both baseline bone mineral density and fracture prevalence. Furthermore, criteria used to define vertebral deformities have varied between studies. In general, however, the reported reduction in fracture has been in the region of 35–50% regardless of the intervention used and thus at present it is not possible to prioritize treatments on the basis of the magnitude of reduction in fracture risk.

Site-specificity

Risk factors for the three main osteoporotic fractures, namely hip, vertebral and distal radius, are overlapping but not identical. In general, a fragility fracture at any site increases the risk of subsequent fractures at other sites;[51,52] ideally, therefore, intervention should protect against all osteoporotic fractures. This may involve beneficial effects not only on bone mineral density at different skeletal sites but also other actions unrelated to bone mass; for example, effects on risk factors for falling and neuromuscular protective mechanisms to such falls. Thus, demonstration of protection against fracture at one skeletal site cannot be assumed to reflect similar effects at other fracture sites.

Of the currently licensed agents, reduced fracture risk at the spine, hip and radius has been demonstrated for only HRT and alendronate. As discussed earlier in this chapter, the evidence for HRT is derived almost exclusively from observational studies whereas that for alendronate is based on adequately powered randomized controlled clinical trials. In the case of raloxifene, although beneficial effects on bone mineral density are seen in both the spine and proximal femur,[53] reduction in fracture risk has been shown only at the spine.[54]

Onset and offset of treatment effect

The minimum duration of therapy required to produce significant protection against fracture is unknown for any of the currently available interventions, although reduction in fracture rate after 12–18 months of therapy has been reported for alendronate and for calcium and vitamin D. The offset of treatment effect is also poorly characterized although, as noted earlier in this chapter, it appears that the skeletal benefits of HRT are not maintained for more than 5 years after withdrawal of treatment and, for the bisphosphonates, bone loss recommences during the first year after treatment is stopped. These observations of the relatively rapid onset and offset of treatment effect, if confirmed, emphasize the potential value of relatively short-term interventions in women with established osteoporosis and provide a strong rationale for targeting high-risk populations for treatment.

Adverse effects

Raloxifene is well tolerated and the only potentially serious adverse effect that has emerged is venous thromboembolism. The increase in relative risk associated with raloxifene therapy is similar to that seen for HRT; although the attributable risk is low in healthy postmenopausal women, both HRT and raloxifene should be avoided in women with a past history of or risk factors for venous thromboembolic disorders. Raloxifene therapy is not associated with an increased risk of gastrointestinal side effects.

Extraskeletal effects

The positioning of HRT and raloxifene depend ultimately on their extraskeletal risks and benefits, particularly with respect to the cardiovascular system, breast, cognitive function and endometrium. Whilst adverse effects of long-term HRT on the breast and endometrium are well documented, effects on coronary heart disease and cognitive function remain to be accurately quantified. In the case of raloxifene, adverse effects on the endometrium are not seen and there is significant protection against breast cancer, at least during the first few years of treatment.[55] However, effects on cardiovascular morbidity and mortality have yet to be established, as have those on cognitive function, and, until the results of prospective studies become available, it is not possible to evaluate accurately the risk–benefit ratio of the long-term use of either intervention.

Current positioning of raloxifene in the prevention of osteoporotic fractures

Raloxifene is a treatment option for postmenopausal women at risk of osteoporotic fracture, particularly women with a low spinal bone mineral density with or without a prevalent vertebral fracture. In view of the lack of evidence for protection against non-vertebral fractures, HRT or bisphosphonates should be regarded as first-line options in women with osteoporosis at non-vertebral sites, particularly the proximal femur. In general, HRT is more appropriate for perimenopausal women because of its beneficial effects on menopausal symptoms whereas bisphosphonates may be preferred by elderly women, in whom tolerance of HRT is often poor.

Raloxifene is a useful option in women with or at risk of osteoporosis who are unable or unwilling to have HRT and are intolerant of bisphosphonates. The evidence for protection against breast cancer is an important consideration in women with a strong fear of this disease who refuse HRT or wish to stop such treatment after a period of 5 years or so. Raloxifene is not suitable for perimenopausal women with active vasomotor menopausal symptoms, in whom HRT remains the treatment of choice.

Future prospects

In the near future, it is likely that the clinical use of SERMs will be limited to osteoporosis and breast cancer, but possible indications in the more distant future include prevention of coronary heart disease and dementia. The potential applications of SERMs are not limited to postmenopausal women but apply also to premenopausal women and men. They include, in the former group, the management of fertility, endometriosis, uterine leiomyoma, and prevention and treatment of premenopausal osteoporosis. In men, the increasing evidence that oestrogen plays a pivotal role in the regulation of bone remodelling provides a strong rationale for the use of SERMs in male osteoporosis; SERMs may also prove useful in the treatment of prostatic cancer, in view of the oestrogen-dependency of these tumours.

The development of SERMs represents a real advance in the management of osteoporosis and, potentially, several other diseases of the postmenopause related to oestrogen status. Advances in our understanding of oestrogen signalling pathways should further elucidate the mechanisms by which tissue specificity may be achieved and thus facilitate the development of agents with specific pharmacological profiles. Furthermore, the lessons learnt from SERMs should also be applicable to other steroid hormones, for example testosterone and glucocorticoids, the therapeutic benefits of which are significantly compromised by adverse effects.

References

1. Compston JE. Prevention and management of osteoporosis: current trends and future prospects. *Drugs* 1997; **53**: 727–35.

2. Compston JE. Mechanisms of drug-induced effects on bone. In: Compston JE (ed). *Osteoporosis.* Royal College of Physicians: London, 1996: 83–95.

3. Kleerekoper M. Fluoride: the verdict is in, but the controversy lingers. *J Bone Miner Res* 1996; **11**: 565–7.

4. Lindsay R, Hart DM, Forrest C, Baird C. Prevention of spinal osteoporosis in oophorectomised women. *Lancet* 1980; **ii**: 1151–3.

5. Christiansen C, Christiensen MS, McNair PL, Hagen C, Stocklund KE, Transbøl I. Prevention of early menopausal bone loss: conducted 2-year. *Eur J Clin Invest* 1980; **10**: 273–9.

6. Hutchinson A, Polansky SM, Feinstein AR. Postmenopausal estrogens protect against fractures of the hip and distal radius: a case control study. *Lancet* 1979; **ii**: 705–9.

7. Weiss NS, Ure CL, Ballard JH, Williams AR, Daling JR, Decreased risk of fractures of the hip and lower forearm with postmenopausal use of estrogens. *N Engl J Med* 1980; **303**: 1195–8.

8. Kiel DP, Felson DT, Anderson JJ, Wilson PWF, Moskowitz MA. Hip fracture and the use of estrogens in postmenopausal women: the Framingham study. *N Engl J Med* 1987; **317**: 1169–74.

9. Schneider DL, Barrett-Connor EL, Morton DJ. Timing of postmenopausal estrogen for optimal bone mineral density. *JAMA* 1997; 277: 543–7.

10. Michaelsson K, Baron JA, Farahmand BY et al. Hormone replacement therapy and risk of hip fracture: a case–control study. *BMJ* 1998; **316**: 1858–63.

11. Quigley MET, Martin PL, Burnier AM, Brooks P. Estrogen therapy arrests bone loss in elderly women. *Am J Obstet Gynecol* 1987; **156**: 1516–23.

12. Colditz GA, Hankinson SE, Hunter DJ et al. The use of estrogens and progestins and the risk of breast cancer in postmenopausal women. *N Engl J Med* 1995; **332**: 1589–93.

13. Collaborative Group on Hormonal Factors in Breast Cancer. Breast cancer and hormone replacement therapy: collaborative reanalysis of data from 51 epidemiological studies of 52,705 women with breast cancer and 108,411 women without breast cancer. *Lancet* 1997; **350**: 1047–59.

14. Daly E, Vessey MP, Hawkins MM, Carson JL, Gough P, Marsh S. Risk of venous thromboembolism in users of hormone replacement therapy. *Lancet* 1996; **348**: 977–80.

15. Jick H, Derby LE, Myers MW, Vasilakis C, Newton KM. Risk of hospital admission for idiopathic venous thromboembolism among users of postmenopausal oestrogens. *Lancet* 1996; **348**: 981–3.

16. Grodstein F, Stampfer JJ, Goldhaber SZ. Prospective study of exogenous hormones and risk of pulmonary embolism. *Lancet* 1996; **348**: 983–7.

17. Gutthann SP, Garcia-Rodriguez LA, Castellsague J, Oliart AD. Hormone replacement therapy and risk of thromboembolism: population based case–control study. *BMJ* 1997; **314**: 796–800

18. Beresford SAA, Weiss NS, Voight LF, McKnight B. Risk of endometrial cancer in

relation to use of oestrogen combined with cyclic progestagen therapy in postmenopausal women. *Lancet* 1997; **349**: 458–61.

19. Grodstein F, Stampfer MJ, Manson JE et al. Postmenopausal estrogen and progestin use and the risk of cardiovascular disease. *N Engl J Med* 1996; **335**: 453–61.

20. Hulley S, Grady D, Bush T et al. Randomized trial of estrogen plus progestin for secondary prevention of coronary heart disease in postmenopausal women. *JAMA* 1998; **280**: 605–13.

21. Henderson VW. The epidemiology of estrogen replacement therapy and Alzheimer's disease. *Neurology* 1997; **48**(suppl 7): S27–S35.

22. Newcomb PA, Storer B. Postmenopausal hormone use and risk of large bowel cancer. *J Natl Cancer Inst* 1995; **87**: 1067–71.

23. Storm T, Kollerup G, Thamsborg G, Genant HK, Sørensen OH. Five years of clinical experience with intermittent cyclical etidronate for postmenopausal osteoporosis. *J Rheumatol* 1996; **23**: 1560–4.

24. Liberman UA, Weiss SR, Bröll J et al. Effect of oral alendronate on bone mineral density and the incidence of fractures in postmenopausal osteoporosis. *N Engl J Med* 1995; **333**: 1437–43.

25. Herd RJM, Balena R, Blake GM, Ryan PJ, Fogelman I. The prevention of early postmenopausal bone loss by cyclical etidronate therapy: a 2-year, double-blind, placebo-controlled study. *Am J Med* 1997; **103**: 92–9.

26. Hosking D, Chilvers CED, Christiansen C et al. Prevention of bone loss with alendronate in postmenopausal women under sixty years of age. *N Engl J Med* 1998; **338**: 485–92.

27. Meunier PJ, Boivin G. Bone mineral density reflects bone mass but also the degree of mineralization of bone: therapeutic implications. *Bone* 1997; **21**: 373–8.

28. Storm T, Thamsborg G, Steiniche T, Genant HK, Sørensen OH. Effect of intermittent cyclical etidronate therapy on bone mass and fracture rate in women with postmenopausal osteoporosis. *N Engl J Med* 1990; **322**: 1265–71.

29. Watts NB, Harris ST, Genant HK et al. Intermittent cyclical etidronate treatment of postmenopausal osteoporosis. *N Engl J Med* 1990; **323**: 72–9.

30. Van Staa TP, Abenhaim L, Cooper C. Use of cyclical etidronate and prevention of non-vertebral fractures. *Br J Rheumatol* 1998; **37**: 87–94.

31. Black DM, Cummings SR, Karpf DB et al. Randomised trial of effect of alendronate on risk of fractures in women with existing vertebral fractures. *Lancet* 1996; **348**: 1535–41.

32. Adachi JD, Bensen WG, Brown J et al. Intermittent etidronate therapy to prevent corticosteroid-induced osteoporosis. *N Engl J Med* 1997; **337**: 382–7.

33. Saag KG, Emkey R, Schnitzer TJ et al. Alendronate for the prevention and treatment of glucocorticoid-induced osteoporosis. *N Engl J Med* 1998; **339**: 292–9.

34. de Groen PC, Lubbe DF, Hirsch LJ. Esophagitis associated with the use of alendronate. *N Engl J Med* 1996; **335**: 1016–21.

35. Meunier PJ, Confavreux E, Tupinon I, Hardouin C, Delmas PD, Balena R. Prevention of early postmenopausal bone loss with cyclical etidronate therapy: a double-blind, placebo-controlled study and 1-year

follow-up. *J Clin Endocrinol Metab* 1997; **82**: 2784–91.

36. Overgaard K, Hansen MA, Jensen SB, Christiansen C. Effect of salcatonin given intranasally on bone mass and fracture rates in established osteoporosis: a dose–response study. *BMJ* 1992; **305**: 556–61.

37. Stock JL, Avioli LV, Baylink DJ et al. Calcitonin-salmon nasal spray reduces the incidence of new vertebral fractures in postmenopausal women: three-year interim results of the PROOF study. *J Bone Miner Res* 1997; **12**(suppl 1): S149.

38. Compston JE. Vitamin D deficiency in the elderly: time for action? *BMJ* 1998; **317**: 1466–7.

39. Chapuy MC, Arlot ME, Duboeuf F et al. Vitamin D3 and calcium to prevent hip fracture in elderly women. *N Engl J Med* 1992; **327**: 1637–42.

40. Dawson-Hughes B, Harris SS, Krall EA, Dallal GE. Effect of calcium and vitamin D supplementation on bone density in men and women 65 years of age and older. *N Engl J Med* 1997; **337**: 670–6.

41. Heikinheimo RJ, Inkovaara JA, Harju EJ. Annual injection of vitamin D and fracture of aged bones. *Calcif Tissue Int* 1992; **51**: 105–10.

42. Lips P, Graafmans WC, Ooms ME, Bezemer PD, Bouter LM. Vitamin D supplementation and fracture incidence in elderly persons: a randomized, placebo-controlled clinical trial. *Ann Intern Med* 1996; **124**: 400–6.

43. Tilyard MW, Spears GFS, Thomson J, Dovey A. Treatment of postmenopausal osteoporosis with calcitriol or calcium. *N Engl J Med* 1992; **326**: 357–62.

44. Orimo H, Shiraki M, Hayashi Y, Hoshino T, Onaya T, Miyazaki S. Effects of 1alpha-hydroxyvitamin D3 on lumbar bone density and vertebral fractures in patients with postmenopausal osteoporosis. *Calcif Tissue Int* 1994; **54**: 370–6.

45. Ott S, Chesnut CH. Calcitriol is not effective in postmenopausal osteoporosis. *Ann Intern Med* 1989; **110**: 267–74.

46. Cumming RG. Calcium intake and bone mass: a quantitative review of the evidence. *Calcif Tissue Int* 1990; **47**: 194–201.

47. Compston JE. The role of vitamin D and calcium supplementation in the prevention of osteoporotic fractures in the elderly. *Clin Endocrinol* 1995; **43**: 393–405.

48. Cumming RG, Nevitt MC. Calcium for prevention of osteoporotic fractures in postmenopausal women. *J Bone Miner Res* 1997; **12**: 1321–9.

49. Riggs BL, Hodgson SF, O'Fallon WM et al. Effect of fluoride treatment on the fracture rate in postmenopausal women with osteoporosis. *N Engl J Med* 1990; **322**: 802–9.

50. Kleerekoper M, Peterson EL, Nelson DA et al. A randomized trial of sodium fluoride as treatment of postmenopausal osteoporosis. *Osteoporos Int* 1991; **1**: 155–61.

51. Ross PD, Genant HK, Davis JW, Miller PD, Wasnich RD. Predicting vertebral fracture incidence from prevalent fractures and bone density among non-black osteoporotic women. *Osteoporos Int* 1993; **3**: 120–6.

52. Wasnich RD, Davis JW, Ross PD. Spine fracture risk is predicted by non-spine fractures. *Osteoporos Int* 1994; **4**: 1–5.

53. Delmas PD, Bjarnason NH, Mitlak BH et al. Effects of raloxifene on bone mineral density, serum cholesterol concentrations and uterine

endometrium in postmenopausal women. *N Engl J Med* 1997; **337**: 1641–7.

54. Ensrud K, Black D, Recker R et al. The effect of 2 and 3 years of raloxifene on vertebral and non-vertebral fractures in postmenopausal women with osteoporosis. *Bone* 1998; **23**: S174.

55. Jordan VC, Glusman JE, Eckert S et al. Incident primary breast cancers are reduced by raloxifene: integrated data from multicenter, double-blind, randomised trials in 12,000 postmenopausal women. *Proc Am Soc Clin Oncol* 1998; **17**: 122a.

Index